10 More Powerful Ideas for Improving Patient Care

Introduction 01

Idea 1 **Harness Creativity to Stimulate Innovative Thinking** 06
The Myth of "Genius" • Directed Creativity • Application of Creative Thinking Tools in Healthcare • Managing the Risk of Innovation

Idea 2 **Give Patients Control** 14
Example: Cincinnati Children's Hospital Medical Center • Example: University of Pittsburgh Medical Center Shadyside

Idea 3 **Use Bundles to Improve Reliability** 21
What Is a Bundle? • Example: The Ventilator Bundle

Idea 4 **Map Out Patterns to Bring About Organizationwide Change** 26
Complex Systems • Five Key Patterns • Facilitating Pattern Mapping • Example: NHS Ophthalmology Service

Idea 5 **Implement Rapid Response Teams** 35
Why Rapid Response Teams? • Acting on Instinct • Design and Implementation of an RRT • Example: Baptist Memorial Hospital

Idea 6 **Reconcile Medications at Every Handoff** 43
Tips for Avoiding Errors at Transition Points • Example: Luther Midelfort Hospital

Idea 7 **Develop Patient Itineraries** 51
Outpatient Flow: The Problem • The Patient Itinerary: A Promising Solution • Example: Two Scenarios Comparing Value-Added Time • Example: Reinier de Graaf Gasthuis

Idea 8 **Measure Bed Turns and Test Changes to Improve Flow** 57
The Hospital Flow Diagnostic Tool • Strategies for Increasing Throughput

Idea 9 **Adopt Acuity-Adjustable Beds and Rooms** 62
Better Design Results in Better Outcomes • Example: Methodist Hospital

Idea 10 **Learn to See** 67
Inattentional Blindness • Task Saturation • Suggestions for Redesigning Processes • Example: SSM Healthcare

About the Authors 72

Acknowledgments 73

Your board, staff, or clients may also benefit from this book's insight. For more information on quantity discounts, contact the Health Administration Press Marketing Manager at (312) 424-9470.

10 09 08 07 06 5 4 3 2 1

Library of Congress Cataloging-in-Publication Data

Bisognano, Maureen A.
10 more powerful ideas for improving patient care / Maureen A. Bisognano and Paul E. Plsek with Dan Schummers.
p. ; cm.
Includes bibliographical references.
ISBN 1-56793-248-7 (alk. paper)
1. Medical care—Quality control. I. Title: Ten more powerful ideas for improving patient care. II. Plsek, Paul E. III. Schummers, Dan. IV. Title.
[DNLM: 1. Quality Assurance, Health Care—methods. 2. Quality Assurance, Health Care—organization & administration. W 84.1 B622z 2005]
RA399.A1B57 2005
362.1'068—dc22

2005052594

The paper used in this publication meets the minimum requirements of American National Standard for Information Sciences-Permanence of Paper for Printed Library Materials, ANSI Z39.48-1984.™

Acquisition manager: Audrey Kaufman; Project manager: Jane Calayag Williams; Cover designer: Trisha Lartz

Health Administration Press
A division of the Foundation of the American College of Healthcare Executives
1 North Franklin Street, Suite 1700
Chicago, IL 60606-4425
(312) 424-2800

Institute for Healthcare Improvement
20 University Road, 7th Floor
Cambridge, MA 02138
(617) 301-4800

Introduction

This is the second book in a series entitled 10 Powerful Ideas for Improving Patient Care, designed to widely share innovations in patient care and operational processes in both inpatient and outpatient settings.

For the first book in this series, authors Jim Reinertsen and Wim Schellekens (2004) pulled together ten ideas from their experience that, if adopted broadly, can begin to change healthcare. Those ideas have been well received, and several have created new care processes and, in some cases, new language as well. The ideas of "moving a big dot" to decrease preventable in-hospital mortality and of "scheduling discharges" (just as admissions are scheduled) are becoming common improvement aims in the United States and abroad.

In this book, we—Maureen Bisognano and Paul Plsek—have joined forces to call attention to ten more promising and innovative ideas and to urge for their adoption across healthcare. Our ideas hold the same promise as those submitted last year, and we invite you to examine them and adopt those that may improve care for patients in your setting.

FINDING GOOD IDEAS AND IMPLEMENTING THEM NOW

We set out to develop this list of ideas for several reasons. First, the work of improvement is challenging and often happens in frustrating isolation. Because we travel widely, we are privileged to see amazing improvements in processes and outcomes in local settings or within defined populations. Promoting the spread of these improvements across all systems would mean that many more patients could benefit from these innovative ideas and better processes. We know from research that best practices typically take 17 years to directly benefit patients at the bedside (Landro 2005). The kinds of improvements detailed in ▸

this book hold promise today, ready for rapid testing and implementation.

Second, many leaders need help in scanning for new ideas that can benefit patients. The proliferation of new science is staggering, and when one considers the need to look into other scientific fields (e.g., reliability science, queuing theory, engineering science, human factors in design), the process can be overwhelming for a single organization. This book includes the results of some of these scans, and as an added benefit most of the ideas presented here have had successful trials in healthcare. Thus, you will find reliable, innovative ideas that have been vetted and used successfully in some local areas and that are referenced so that your team can follow up for further information.

SPREADING CHANGES THROUGHOUT THE ORGANIZATION

In their book, Reinertsen and Schellekens describe a leadership model that has helped healthcare leaders to make faster improvements. Developed by Tom Nolan (2000) and expanded by the Institute for Healthcare Improvement (IHI) (Reinertsen et al. 2003), this leadership model is shown in Figure A.

In this book, we suggest an additional model to support your senior team's efforts—a Framework for Spread shown in Figure B (on page 4). This model was developed at IHI through collaboration among Tom Nolan, Kevin Nolan, colleagues at Associates in Process Improvement, senior fellows at IHI, and IHI director Marie Schall (Nolan et al. 2005).

A Framework for Spread has helped us plan and execute the diffusion of new ideas and new performance levels, both within an organization and between similar systems. Healthcare leaders can often find points of excellence in parts of the hospital or clinic setting, but they may rely on local leaders or improvement teams to spread these best practices. Donald Berwick, M.D., president and chief executive officer of IHI, often calls this the "6-West" problem: Leaders can find and celebrate performance excellence somewhere within the system, but they cannot promise the same level of experience in clinical care across the entire system—that is, they cannot ensure that the successes in the hypothetical "6-West" ward make it to the "6-East" ward. In our experience, complete and reliable spread across all units happens only when leaders drive the diffusion,

Figure A. Institute for Healthcare Improvement Leadership Model

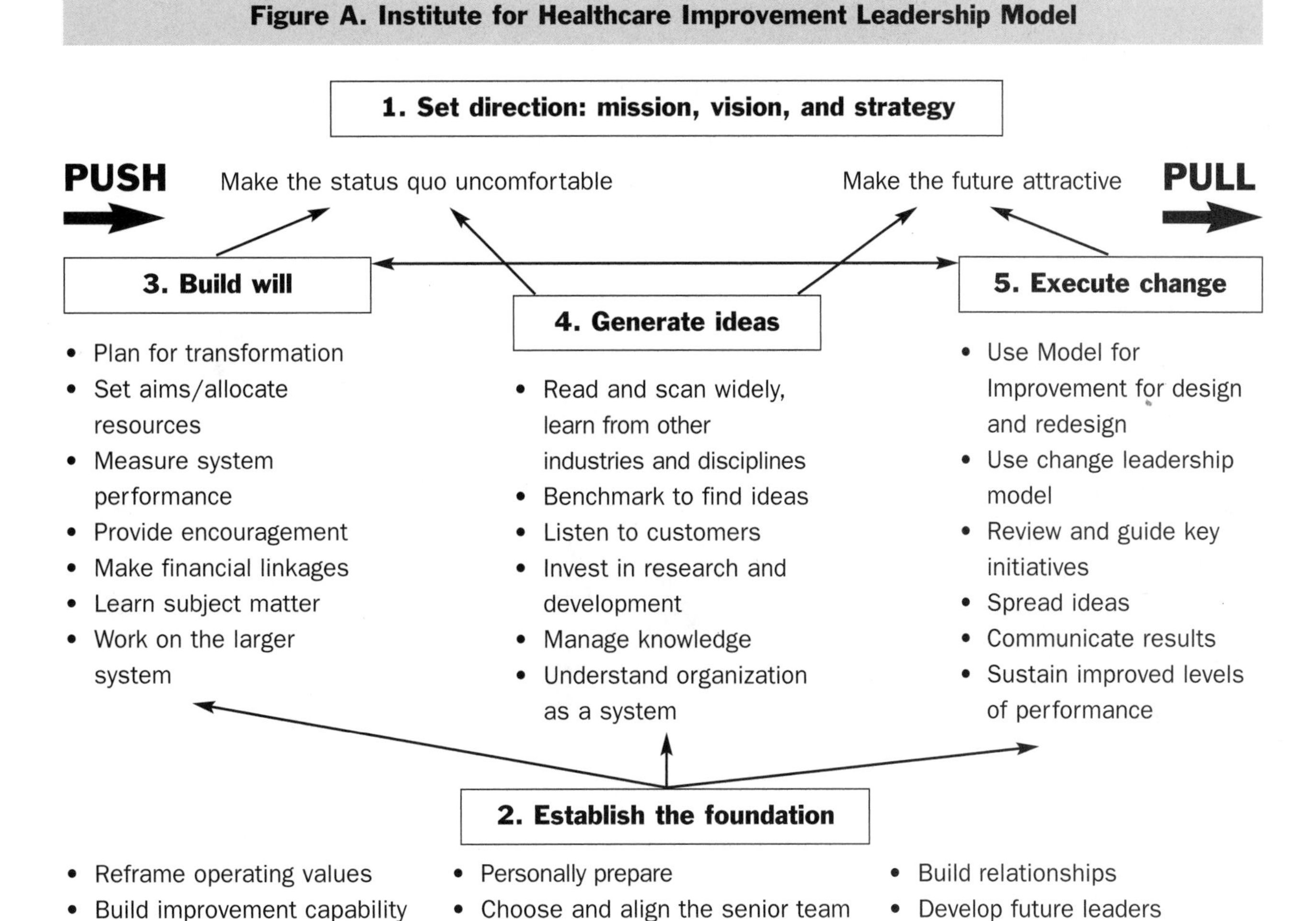

Source: Reprinted with permission from Institute for Healthcare Improvement, Cambridge, Massachusetts.

often using a model such as a Framework for Spread.

We hope that this framework, in conjunction with the ideas presented in this book, will help get you started with or accelerate your improvement work.

WHY THESE IDEAS?

As you read through the book, you are likely to ask, "Why these ideas?" We—a leader of a healthcare quality improvement organization and an improvement and innovation

Figure B. A Framework for Spread

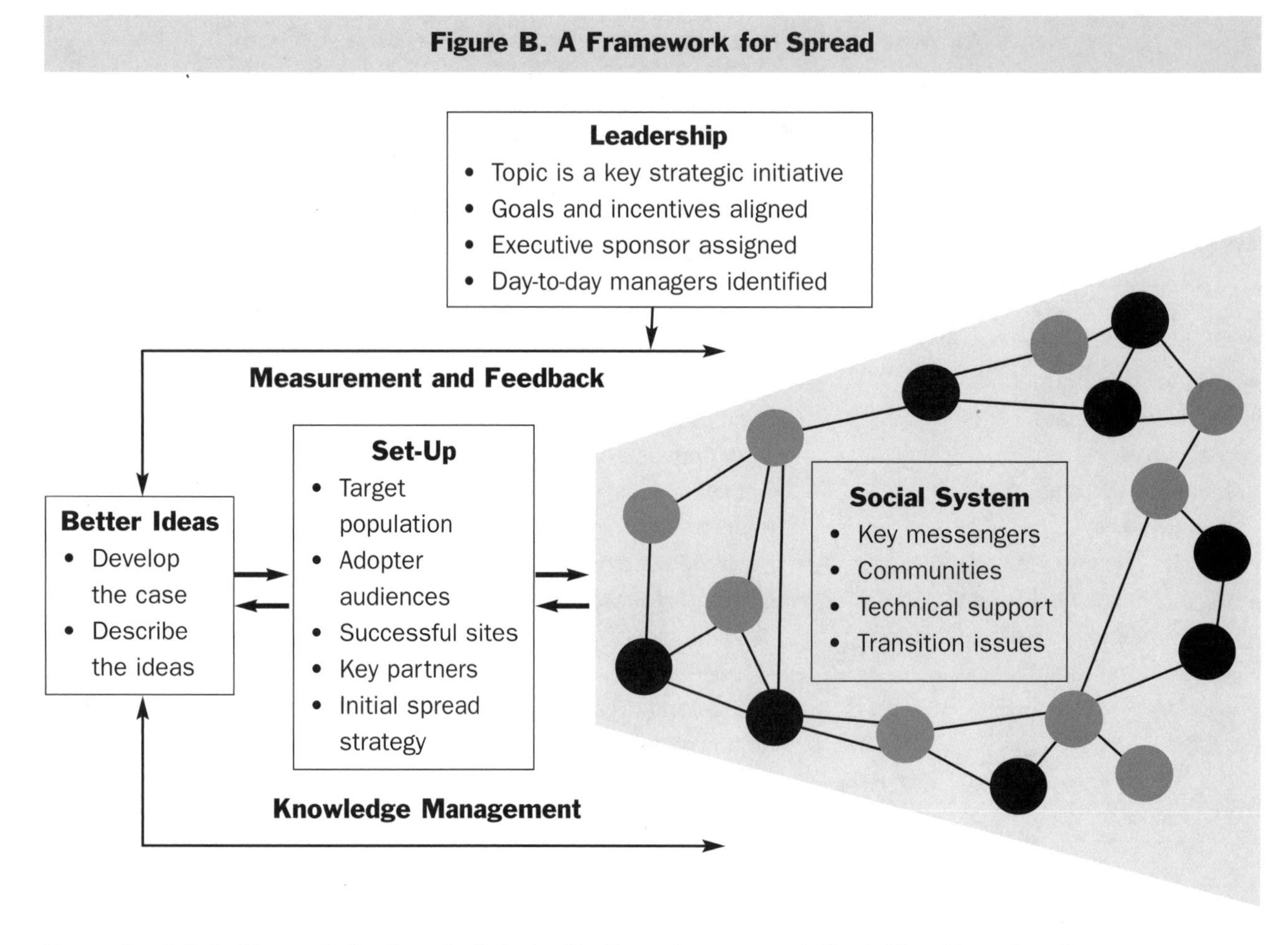

Source: Reprinted with permission from Institute for Healthcare Improvement, Cambridge, Massachusetts.

consultant, respectively—come across hundreds of exciting and promising ideas. Incorporating the best of these ideas into our work is integral to our mission of quality improvement in healthcare. To determine which ideas would be included in this volume, we asked ourselves these questions:

- Would we want to use this idea in our own organizations?
- Does this idea have appeal for leaders at multiple levels in an organization, not just the CEO?
- Does this idea have appeal across multiple clinical and professional disciplines?

- Does this idea have the potential to truly transform things, to go beyond merely incremental improvement?
- Is this idea being used?

Ideas that passed the test—that is, for which all answers to these questions were "yes"—became prime candidates for inclusion.

HOW TO USE THIS BOOK

Ten ideas are explored in this book, each with its own chapter. A chapter provides a description of the idea, an example of the idea in practice, and the results that have been achieved with the application of the idea.

Leaders may use this book in a variety of ways. Some may read it straight through, getting an overview of all ten ideas and thinking broadly about how the ideas may fit into their organizational strategy. Others may want to zero-in on the ideas that hold particular relevance for their organizations. It is not necessary to read the book sequentially, as all the ideas intersect in one way or another and each idea is understandable on its own. We encourage readers to choose whatever sequence interests them.

Above all, our hope is that these ideas lead to *action*: Pick one, or two, or all ten, and then try them out. Ask yourself, as we are fond of saying at IHI, "What can I do by next Tuesday?"

REFERENCES

Landro, L. 2005. "Informed Patient: Healthcare Quality Programs Under Fire." *The Wall Street Journal* July 6, page D1.

Nolan, T. 2000. "A Primer on Leading Improvement in Healthcare." Presented at the 5th European Forum on Quality Improvement in Health Care, Amsterdam, March 24.

Nolan, K., M. Schall, F. Erb, and T. Nolan. 2005. "Using a Framework for Spread: The Case of Patient Access in the Veterans Health Administration." *Joint Commission Journal on Quality and Safety* 31 (6): 339–47.

Reinertsen, J. L., M. Bisognano, L. Provost, T. Nolan, and W. Rupp. 2003. "Leading to Perfection: A Model of Leadership for Transformation." White paper. Cambridge, MA: Institute for Healthcare Improvement.

Reinertsen, J. L., and W. Schellekens. 2004. *10 Powerful Ideas for Improving Patient Care.* Chicago: Health Administration Press.

IDEA 1

Harness Creativity to Stimulate Innovative Thinking

"The challenge is to bring the full potential benefit of effective health care to all ... this challenge demands a readiness to think in radically new ways about how to deliver health care services."

—*Crossing the Quality Chasm* (Institute of Medicine)

EXTRA! EXTRA! Healthcare professionals are really creative! It's about time that we discovered and appreciated the creativity of our staff, physicians, and leaders. The Institute of Medicine (IOM) suggests that we are not going to cross the "quality chasm" until we are ready to think in radically new ways.

Based on advances in medical, surgical, and diagnostic technologies, a general impression in society is that healthcare is a highly innovative industry. But the ▸

sad fact is that we routinely take the latest twenty-first century technology and embed it in our service delivery process, which has not fundamentally changed since the 1950s or 1960s. A healthcare consumer still has to get an appointment, check in with the receptionist, sit in the waiting room, read the magazines, and wait to be called into the doctor's office. It is about time for this process to go through some rethinking.

Of course, there have been important improvements in service delivery using traditional methods. But while efficiency and flow have improved, the same basic patterns (or "just the way we do it in healthcare") persist: appointments, waiting, and going through lower-cost resources before getting to higher-cost resources (e.g., from receptionist to nurse to doctor). To *truly* innovate, we must alter these fundamental process design patterns. We need tools that will enable us not only to critically examine the outward manifestations of a problem (e.g., waiting time) but also to challenge the underlying thinking that contributes to, if not causes, the problem (e.g., if it were suddenly against the law to have a waiting area, how would we handle patient intake?). This requires that we augment the traditional methods of problem solving and incremental improvement with new methods for stimulating innovative thinking (see Figure C).

THE MYTH OF "GENIUS"

The myth is that creativity is a special gift of genius that is given only to a few people. In reality, a vast number of studies on innovation suggest that everyone is capable of thinking creatively, but some of us have forgotten how or have not engaged in it for quite a while.

At its heart, creativity involves connecting and rearranging knowledge. A great example of this concept of taking things that already exist and putting them together in a new way is the invention of the Ziploc® storage bag. Imagine the person who went up to the new product development committee back in the 1960s and said, "I've got this great idea: Put zippers on plastic bags!" Laughter was the likely response. That surprise, that initial laughter is a function—and failing—of organizational culture. In a typical meeting in which real problems in healthcare are being addressed, a surprising idea that makes everyone laugh can get dismissed immediately. But those ideas are often the most creative

Figure C. Levels of Improvement and Change

Level	Goal	Underlying Mental Models
Problem solving	Return to prior performance or meet standard	Untouched
Incremental improvement	Better performance	Untouched
Redesign	Dramatically better performance	Several changes, most remain
Rethinking	Dramatically better performance; wow!; redefine the way	Everything is on the table for questioning

things said during the entire meeting.

Creativity is the production of new, often surprising ideas that others judge to be useful. You do not have to be a genius to be creative. You just need an environment in which people give themselves permission to think flexibly.

DIRECTED CREATIVITY

How do we harness the creativity of healthcare professionals and use it to address real problems? One answer is to use the methods and tools of *directed creativity*. Simply defined, directed creativity is the purposeful generation of new ideas in a given topic area, followed up by deliberate effort to implement some of those ideas. It is creativity on demand.

When we need a creative idea, telling ourselves and others to "think harder," "suspend judgment" (as in brainstorming), or "be playful" does little good. While these suggestions are indeed helpful, they fail to provide a new direction for thinking. Thus, we may find that we are only able to come up with small variations on the mental patterns we already have (e.g., ways to reduce waiting, rather than fundamentally new ways to handle patient intake if waiting areas were outlawed).

Directed creativity involves using specific techniques to perceive things in a fresh way, break free from the current patterns stored in memory, make novel associations among concepts stored in memory, and use judgment to develop rather than immediately reject new ideas.

Three Principles of Directed Creativity

Underlying the hundreds of tools in the creativity literature are three simple principles: attention, escape, and movement.

To begin creative thinking, we need to direct our *attention* to things that we normally ignore or take for granted—for example, a clinic must have a waiting area, the patient has to come to the hospital or clinic if he or she wants healthcare, or the patient has to park his or her car and then come in for service. Put another way, for us to be able to think "outside the box," we must first notice that we are *in* a box in the way we think about things in healthcare.

To continue thinking creatively, we must mentally *escape* the trap of "that's just how it is" mind-set. We can trigger this mental escape by considering a challenging scenario: What would we do if waiting areas in healthcare organizations were outlawed? We may also temporarily approach the problem scenario from another point of view: Banks no longer require customers to come to a branch for service; what can we learn from that? Fast-food restaurants and dry cleaning stores do not make customers get out of their car; what healthcare services can we offer using a drive-through window?

We bet that the suggestion of the drive-through window in a healthcare facility made you laugh. This is the type of mental trap that we must escape, and it emphasizes the importance of mental *movement* to innovative thinking. The suggestion seems silly at first, but rather than reject it, we should allow our minds to continue moving and brainstorm a list of services that may be offered in a drive-through capacity. For example, the drive-through window may be used for dropping off lab samples or paperwork, getting a quick referral to a dermatologist for a skin discoloration, doing a quick triage that will send nonurgent patients to other specialty clinics, or getting a flu shot.

You may still be laughing at these suggestions, but if you keep moving in your thinking, you may develop an innovative service delivery concept.

For example, Monadnock Community Hospital in New Hampshire, Veterans Medical Center in Texas, and the Loma Linda University Medical Center and Children's Hospital in California are among the healthcare organizations that are successfully giving flu shots in drive-through clinics.

APPLICATION OF CREATIVE THINKING TOOLS IN HEALTHCARE

These three simple principles open the way to the development of a large number of directed creativity methods. The transfer of the concept of a drive-through window from the fast-food industry into healthcare is an example of a directed creativity tool called *mental benchmarking*. Typically, healthcare organizations visit other healthcare organizations to "benchmark" performance and services. This activity involves attention and movement in thinking, but it lacks escape. Selecting another industry at random, and thinking about how they provide service, provides the mental escape for truly creative ideas to emerge.

The following tools are simply various combinations of practical ways to focus attention, escape the current reality, and continue mental movement.

Random picture. This technique involves escape by looking through randomly selected pictures that have nothing to do with healthcare. Here, we focus attention on the pictures and then move on to brainstorm how the concepts in the images may apply to the healthcare problem at hand. For example, a team in the NHS Modernisation Agency in the United Kingdom that was looking for creative ideas in public health promotion focused on a picture of a refrigerator. The team then generated the idea of creating a "refrigerator audit" checklist that school children could take home to explore with their parents whether the family's diet was a healthy one.

In another example, an emergency services group in a major urban hospital in the United States that was exploring how they might cope with a terrorist attack focused on a picture of a man in a hammock. The group is now working with a vendor to create emergency care beds that can be quickly hung on wall supports in bunk-bed fashion, allowing the department to rapidly double its bed capacity.

Scene modification. This tool involves paying attention to the details in a common scene, allowing escape from the current use or constraints of such items. This process then moves on to brainstorming to come up with creative ideas. This tool was used by managers in a large HMO that was introducing copays who were concerned about the interaction between staff and members at check-in. Among the items that the managers imagined in this typical scene were a member's wallet with multiple cards in it and a calendar on the wall. This led to the idea of developing a "gift of health" card that can be purchased for another person who, in turn, may only use the card for copays at the HMO. Note that the group could have come up with this idea using the mental benchmarking technique or by seeing such gift cards at video rental stores. It does not matter how the creative mental connections come about; what matters is that they do come about.

Breaking the rules. This was the method that the Institute of Medicine committee that wrote the *Crossing the Quality Chasm* report used to foster creative thinking. This tool begins with sharing narrative stories of patients' common experiences in the healthcare system and observing the apparent "rules" in the system. For example, we notice that care is provided on the basis of visits—that is, if people want healthcare, they have to go to the doctor's office. What if we escaped that notion and instead think, "people can't go to the office." Mental movement leads to the observation that healthcare involves the exchange of information. An e-mail, telephone, or an online (Internet) consultation with a doctor is an innovative idea, precisely because it breaks the implicit current rule that care can be received only with an office visit. To be innovative, we have to pay attention to the current, implicit process design rules, escape them, and move in our thinking.

Methods such as these are currently being systematically incorporated into the quality improvement toolkit of pioneering healthcare organizations such as the Virginia Mason Medical Center in Seattle, Washington, and the National Health Service in the United Kingdom. They are also being used in grant-supported efforts to redesign well-child care and the addiction treatment system.

MANAGING THE RISK OF INNOVATION

Note that a truly innovative idea—something that has never been tried before in healthcare—is always associated with a certain risk. It may not work or, worse, it may actually cause harm. All creative ideas should be subjected to a set of questions like those shown in Figure D. The amount of effort devoted to what the innovation literature calls "enhancement" will depend on the inherent risk associated with the idea. For example, the potential risks associated with the drive-through flu shot idea deserve a good deal of attention.

Note also that the testability and prototyping question in Figure D naturally leads to the traditional quality improvement model of the Plan-Do-Study-Act (PDSA) cycle. Innovative ideas can be tested and scaled up in the same way as any other idea that may come from evidence or best-practice investigations.

The keys to innovative thinking are captured in the following mental actions:

Figure D. Enhancing Creative Ideas

- *Shaping:* How can we modify the idea to address objections that would otherwise cause rejection?
- *Tailoring:* Can we modify the idea to even better fit our needs?
- *Strengthening:* How can we increase the power or value of the idea?
- *Reinforcing:* What can we do about weak points?
- *Looking toward implementation:* What can we do to the idea to enhance the probability of implementation? Who must be involved?
- *Comparison to current practice:* How does the idea compare to what it is replacing? Should we do further enhancement, expand, or scale back the idea?
- *Potential faults or defects:* What can possibly go wrong with this idea? What can we do?
- *Consequences:* What are the immediate and long-term consequences of putting the idea into action?
- *Testability and prototyping:* How can we try the idea on a small scale?
- *Preevaluation:* How can we further modify the idea to meet the needs of those who will evaluate it next?

- Pay attention to everything around us, especially our patterns of thinking.
- Escape the confines of our current thinking on a topic, premature judgment, and the desire to maintain the status quo.
- Move flexibly in our thinking to explore how we may connect our problem to things we already know.
- Harvest and enhance the best ideas, with attention to risk.
- Test a few ideas through small-scale tests of change (PDSA cycles).

WHERE TO LEARN MORE

Corrigan, J. M., M. S. Donaldson, and L. T. Kohn (eds.). 2001. *Crossing the Quality Chasm: A New Health System for the 21st Century*. Washington, DC: National Academies Press, Institute of Medicine.
Plsek, P. E. 1999. "Innovative Thinking for the Improvement of Medical Systems." *Annals of Internal Medicine* 131 (6): 438–44.

Plsek, P. E. 2002. "Building a Mind Set of Service Excellence." *Family Practice Management* 9 (4): 41–46.

To learn more about directed creativity, please visit http://www.DirectedCreativity.com.

To see more examples of directed creativity tools that are being used in the National Health Service in the United Kingdom, please visit http://www.content.modern.nhs.uk/cmsWISE/Cross+Cutting+Themes/Innovation/Tools/Creativity+Tools.htm.

To learn more about PDSA cycles and testing changes, please visit http://www.ihi.org/IHI/Topics/Improvement/ImprovementMethods/HowToImprove/testingchanges.htm.

IDEA 2

Give Patients Control

Care has often become centered not around the needs of patients, but around the needs of the system itself.

The Institute of Medicine's (2001) report, *Crossing the Quality Chasm*, established the following six "aims for improvement":

1. Safety
2. Effectiveness
3. Patient-centeredness
4. Timeliness
5. Efficiency
6. Equity

This chapter focuses on the third aim: patient-centeredness.

The report elaborated on the patient-centeredness goals, calling for healthcare systems that ▸

- respect patients' values, preferences, and expressed needs;
- coordinate and integrate care across boundaries of the system;
- provide the information, communication, and education that people need and want; and
- guarantee physical comfort, emotional support, and the involvement of family and friends.

While these characteristics of care are widely accepted, they are not always well implemented. As the healthcare system has grown more complex and fragmented, and as providers feel more pressure to see more patients in less time, care has often become centered not around *the needs of patients*, but around *the needs of the system itself.*

Care that is patient-centered considers patients' cultural traditions, personal preferences and values, family situations, and lifestyles. It makes the patient the leader of a multidisciplinary care team, putting responsibility for important aspects of self-care and monitoring in the patient's hands and giving the patient the tools and support needed to carry out that responsibility.

Unlike the other emerging approaches discussed in this book, the idea of giving patients more control does not require a great deal of explanation. Thus, rather than expanding on this idea, we provide the following two examples of hospitals that are making the decision to give patients more control over their own care.

EXAMPLE: CINCINNATI CHILDREN'S HOSPITAL MEDICAL CENTER

At Cincinnati Children's Hospital Medical Center in Ohio, the historical method of taking care of patients with diabetes was to give them a prescription for insulin and have them adjust their diet accordingly. In the past, diabetes patients changed their diet, took their insulin at the prescribed rate and dosage every day, and then had their blood sugar tested. Today, Cincinnati Children's is testing a new theory in caring for diabetics. Instead of adjusting the patient's diet to the insulin, the hospital tells the patient, "Eat your normal diet, eat a healthy diet, and *then* test and adjust your insulin to that diet."

A debate arose among hospital physicians over which method was better. So they conducted a trial in which they asked the patient and his or her family (spouse, partner, children, or parents), "Which process would you rather follow: Do you want to *adjust your diet to the insulin,* or do you want to eat your normal diet and *adjust your insulin to the diet?*"

What doctors found was that patients did better by selecting the diabetic protocol that they felt more comfortable with and then adopting it in their own way (see Figure E). The intervening variable here was not one protocol or the other; it was *choice.* When the hospital allowed patients to choose, *all* patients' hemoglobin A1c's dropped below the previous levels.

EXAMPLE: UNIVERSITY OF PITTSBURGH MEDICAL CENTER SHADYSIDE

This example involves the University of Pittsburgh Medical Center

Figure E. Cincinnati Children's Hospital Medical Center: Effect of Choice of Treatment on Average Hemoglobin A1c

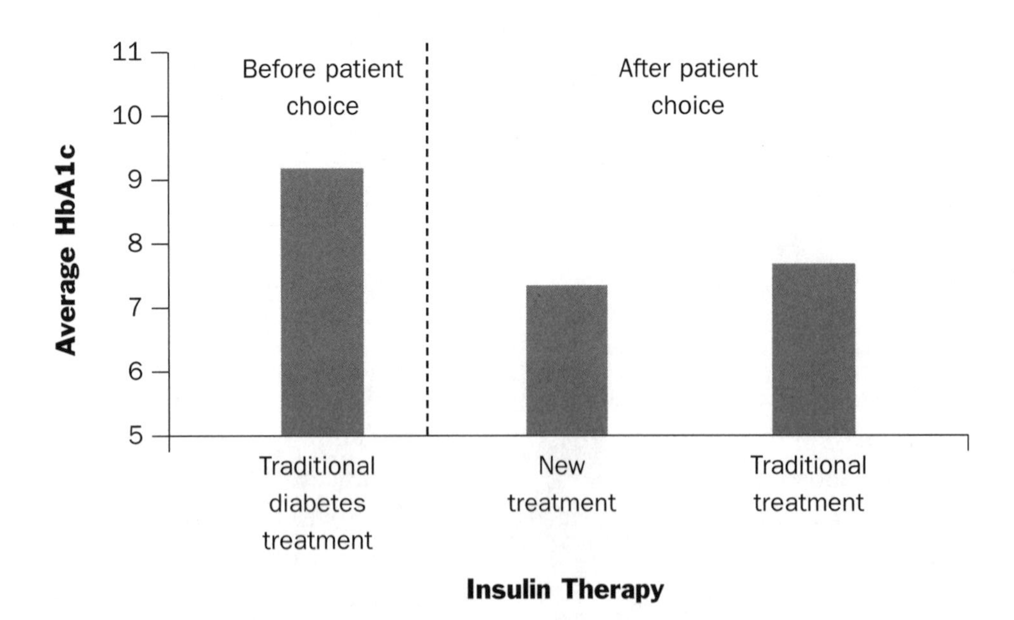

Source: Reprinted with permission from Cincinnati Children's Hospital Medical Center, Cincinnati, Ohio.

(UPMC) Shadyside's examination of a process that was causing a lot of consternation and unreliability: the dietary process. UPMC decided to try letting its patients control their own diet. The hospital changed the process pretty dramatically and sought both to improve clinical outcomes for nutrition education and to reduce the complexity of the dietary process. Note the difference between the traditional process (see Figure F) and the new process (see Figure G).

In the patient-controlled diet process, patients order their meals and the provider checks in with them to see whether the chosen food complies with the guidelines of the diet. The trigger for a provider's visit to the patient is when the menu

Figure F. UPMC Shadyside: Traditional Dietary Process

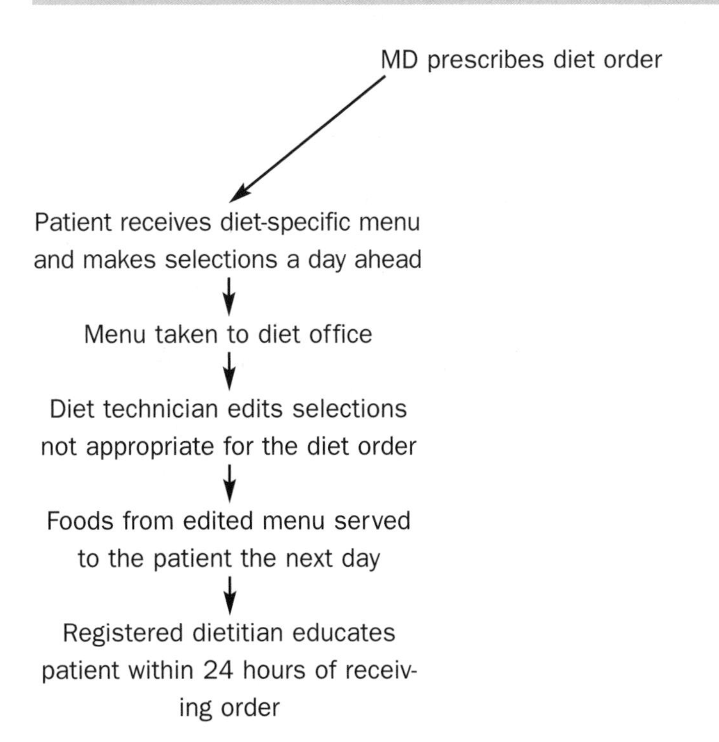

Source: Reprinted with permission from the University of Pittsburgh Medical Center Shadyside, Pittsburgh, Pennsylvania.

Figure G. UPMC Shadyside: Patient-Controlled Liberalized Diet

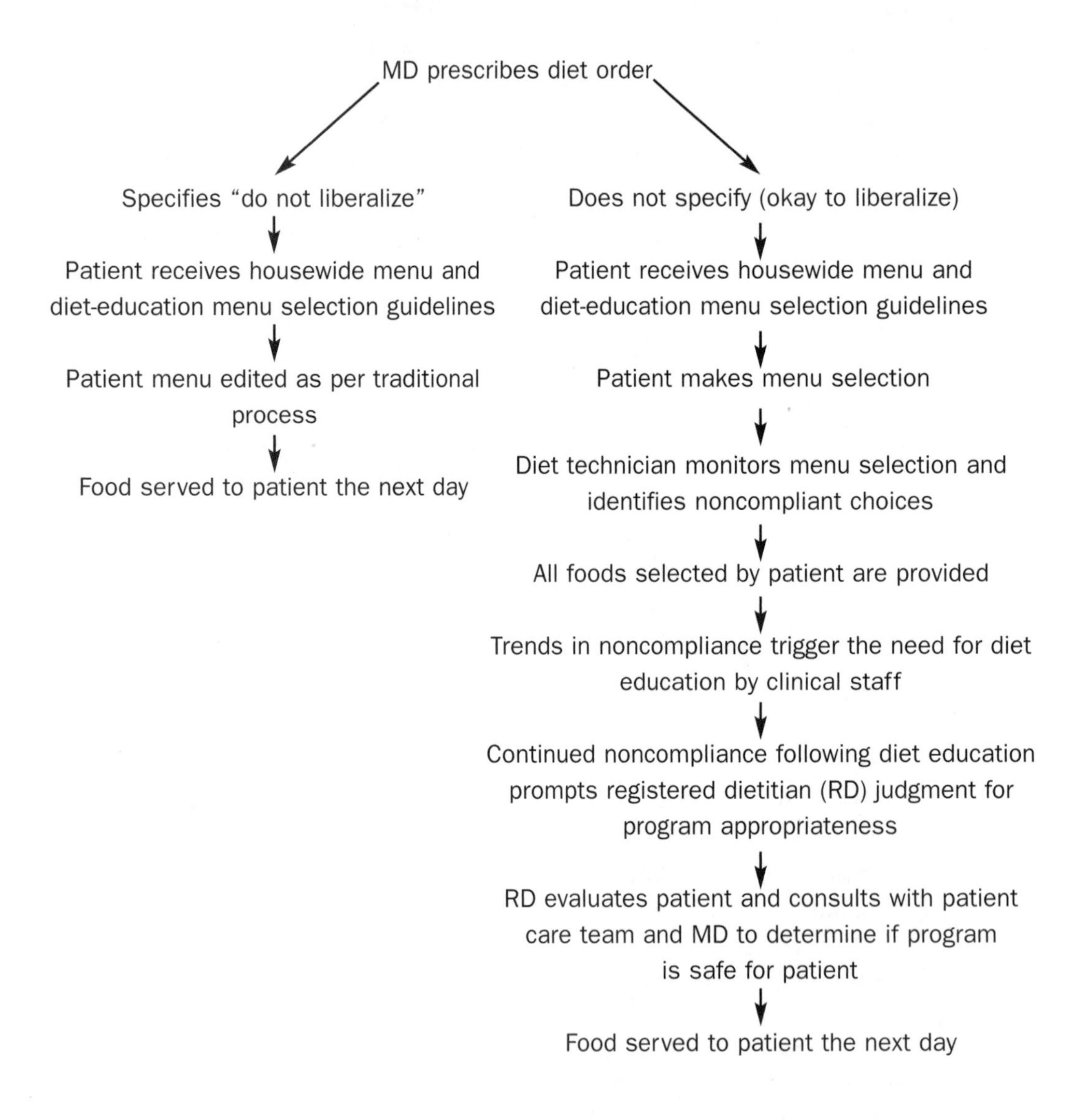

Source: Reprinted with permission from the University of Pittsburgh Medical Center Shadyside, Pittsburgh, Pennsylvania.

selection is not compliant. However, instead of simply changing the diet tray, the provider uses this opportunity to educate the patient about nutrition. The provider talks with the patient about food choices and how to adjust the diet more sensibly. The results of the new dietary process at UPMC are as follows:

- A 58 percent increase in the number of patients who rated the food service as "exceeds or greatly exceeds expectations" (Patient satisfaction after six months of implementation)
- 25 percent increase in the number of patients who consumed 75 percent or more of the food on their trays (Patient intake after six months of implementation)
- 10 percent increase in the number of patients selecting food items appropriate for their prescribed diet (Patient compliance monitored during initial roll-out)
- 22 percent increase in the number of patient educational opportunities for diet instruction as a result of implementing a new educational screening process via menu-selection monitoring (Education interventions monitored during initial roll-out)

Anyone familiar with patient complaints about food service will appreciate the significance of the increase in patient satisfaction. Because many elderly patients lose nutritional ground during their hospitalization, the patient intake result from the modified process is also very encouraging. The improvement in patient compliance is linked to early educational interventions, follow-up and tracking, and giving the patients informed control of their diet.

UPMC observed indirect findings as well. Initially, there was staff resistance, as turning over control to patients was not easy for staff. There were concerns about patient safety as well, but they did not prove to be true. UPMC found the new process to be cost-effective. This process improvement resulted in staff members learning new skills, specifically in the area of working with patients to make their own care decisions.

WHERE TO LEARN MORE

Corrigan, J. M., M. S. Donaldson, and L. T. Kohn (eds.). 2001. *Crossing the Quality Chasm: A New Health System for the 21st Century*. Washington, DC: National Academies Press, Institute of Medicine.

Holman, H. 2004. "Chronic Disease—The Need for a New Clinical Education." *JAMA* 292 (9): 1057–59.

Institute for Healthcare Improvement. "Involving Patients in Redesigning Care." Video within the seven-part "Pursuing Perfection in Health Care" motivational series of videotapes. Please visit http://www.ihi.org/IHI/Products/Video/InvolvingPatientsinRedesigningCareVideo.htm.

IDEA 3

Use Bundles to Improve Reliability

All or none

Nosocomial pneumonia is the leading cause of death from hospital-acquired infections. In one study, ventilator-associated pneumonia (VAP) accounted for 60 percent of all deaths caused by hospital-associated infections (Tablan et al. 2004). Hospital mortality for patients who develop VAP is 46 percent, compared to 32 percent for patients who do not develop VAP (Ibrahim et al. 2001). VAP can prolong a stay in the intensive care unit (ICU) by an average of 4.3 to 6.1 days and can prolong a stay in the hospital by 4 to 9 days. These prolonged stays can produce excess costs of approximately $40,000 per patient (Tablan et al. 2004). These numbers paint a grim picture, to be sure, but not a hopeless one.

At IHI's National Forum on Quality Improvement in Health Care in December 2004, IHI's CEO Dr. Donald Berwick announced the 100,000 Lives Campaign—a national initiative to prevent 100,000 avoidable deaths in hospitals by June 14, 2006. At ▸

the heart of this campaign are six interventions that, if adopted by hospitals as standard practices, can dramatically reduce mortality. Of these six interventions, two involve the use of so-called "bundles." One of these bundles is aimed at preventing hazardous central-line-associated bloodstream infections. The other is aimed at preventing VAP, a condition whose intervention is discussed in this chapter as an example of the promising results of the emerging bundles approach.

WHAT IS A BUNDLE?

Key care processes typically involve several steps to facilitate a comprehensive, safe, and reliable outcome. What distinguishes a bundle from a simple set of individual processes?

1. *A bundle is evidence-based as opposed to "customary."* Too often in healthcare, staff use processes and practices simply because "that's the way things have always been done." However, it has become clear that using processes and practices that are evidence-based—have been scientifically tested and proven to positively affect outcomes—is a much more reliable method of providing excellent care.

2. *A bundle is composed of interrelated processes.* In terms of both implementation and measurement, the concept of bundles is all or none. In the past, reliability was measured by the rate of implementation of individual processes. But what bundles demand is composite reliability—that is, *only when each and every individual process within the bundle is carried out is the overall process considered complete or successful.*

3. *The number of elements in a given bundle needs to be small.* This trait results from the all-or-none mentality. When fewer processes exist, each process is more likely to be implemented in every instance, thereby increasing reliability.

4. *Key processes of a bundle must be carried out in the same space and within a set time.* This characteristic is also linked to the all-or-none mentality. For a bundle to achieve its goal of increased reliability, the individual processes that have been bundled together must occur in the same space (in an ICU, for example) and within an established, relatively short period of time. If the space and time are too dissimilar, then the power of the all-or-none measurement gets diluted or even lost as a strong team- and infrastructure-building component.

This last point highlights one of

the most encouraging "side effects" of bundles: They have benefits not only for the patient but also for the caregivers. Bundles help to identify failures and point out places where processes are flawed or people are not trained well enough. Once those failures have been identified, thinking about new ways to work together can begin. As a result of the use of bundles, we frequently see teamwork and cooperation improving in a dramatic way. We are starting to see physicians and nurses making patient rounds together and talking about daily goals with the patient. This kind of teamwork and communication improvement is just as important as the clinical improvements.

In summary, a bundle is a grouping of evidence-based processes with proximate time and space characteristics that, when performed collectively, can have an enhanced effect on an outcome. What kind of outcome might this be? One example is a significant reduction in mortality related to VAP.

EXAMPLE: THE VENTILATOR BUNDLE

The ventilator bundle consists of four elements:

1. Elevation of the head of the bed to between 30 and 45 degrees
2. Daily "sedation vacation" and assessment of readiness to extubate
3. Peptic ulcer disease (PUD) prophylaxis
4. Deep venous thrombosis (DVT) prophylaxis

While only elevation of the head of the bed and sedation vacations have been shown to have an effect on VAP, all four interventions are backed by medical evidence and independently affect patient mortality and morbidity (Resar et al. 2005).

In more general terms, the ventilator bundle is a package of evidence-based interventions that, when implemented together for all patients on mechanical ventilation, has resulted in dramatic reductions in the incidence of VAP. How dramatic are these results?

Consider the example of Our Lady of Lourdes Hospital in Binghamton, New York. Using the ventilator bundle, this hospital went 290 days (from March 2004 to January 2005) without a single case of VAP. Although the hospital experienced one VAP case in January 2005, it had gone an additional 48 days with a VAP rate of zero (data as of February 28, 2005). The Y-axis in Figure H shows the hospital's VAP rate per 1,000 ventilator days.

Figure H. Our Lady of Lourdes Hospital: Ventilator-Associated Pneumonia Rate

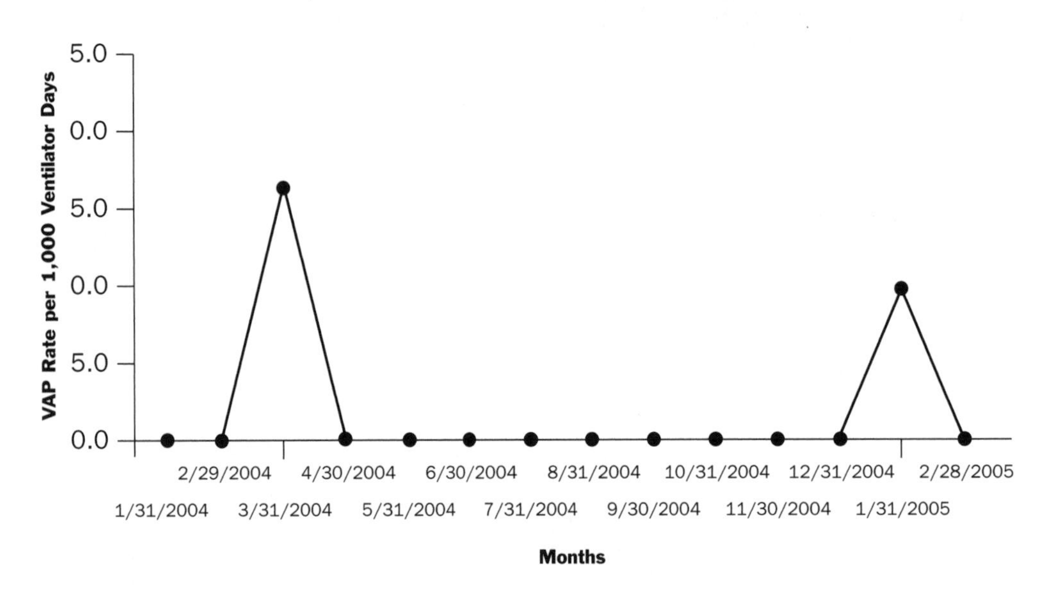

Source: Reprinted with permission from Our Lady of Lourdes Hospital, Binghamton, New York.

WHERE TO LEARN MORE

Information on the scientific basis for the four elements of the ventilator bundle can be found in the 100,000 Lives Campaign section of IHI's web site: http://www.ihi.org/IHI/Programs/Campaign/Campaign.htm?TabId = 2#Prevent%20Ventilator-Associated%20Pneumonia.

Baptist Memorial Hospital in Memphis, Tennessee, implemented several best practices in the ICU, including the ventilator bundle. The hospital achieved a reduction in the incidence of VAP and a decline in ICU length of stay. See the story at http://www.ihi.org/IHI/Topics/Improvement/ImprovementMethods/ImprovementStories/MemberReportRealChangeLeadstoImprovedICUPatientCare.htm.

More detailed information about the ventilator bundle can be found on IHI's web site: http://www.ihi.org/IHI/Programs/Campaign/Campaign.htm?TabId=2#Prevent%20VentilatorAssociated%20Pneumonia.

REFERENCES

Ibrahim, E. H., L. Tracy, C. Hill, V. J. Fraser, and M. H. Kollef. 2001. "The Occurrence of Ventilator-Associated Pneumonia in a Community Hospital: Risk Factors and Clinical Outcomes." *Chest* 120 (2): 555–61.

Resar, R., P. Pronovost, C. Haraden, T. Simmonds, T. Rainey, and T. Nolan. 2005. "Using a Bundle Approach to Improve Ventilator Care Processes and Reduce Ventilator-Associated Pneumonia." *Joint Commission Journal on Quality and Patient Safety* 31 (5): 243–48.

Tablan, O. C., L. J. Anderson, R. Besser, C. Bridges, and R. Hajjeh. 2004. "Guidelines for Preventing Health-Care-Associated Pneumonia, 2003: Recommendations of CDC and the Healthcare Infection Control Practices Advisory Committee." *Morbidity and Mortality Weekly Report* 53 (RR-3): 1–179.

IDEA 4

Map Out Patterns to Bring About Organizationwide Change

"Working on patterns was like letting the genie out of the bottle. If we hadn't looked at patterns, we wouldn't have achieved what we did—because all that baggage was getting in the way."

—Director of Service Modernisation, NHS Trust, United Kingdom

While traditional improvement methods have yielded impressive results, it is clear that large-scale change—organizationwide change —in healthcare is an elusive goal. Why do organizational transformation efforts tend to fall short of expectations? Just as one of the aims of directed creativity (see Idea 1) is to focus attention on unchallenged mental models that underlie, and often undermine, creativity, this chapter focuses ▸

on the tensions among the various parts of a complex system that often undermine organizationwide change.

Our hypothesis is that the inability of a system to reach its aspirations (despite good, traditional improvement work) is largely the result of poorly understood and poorly managed tensions within a complex system.

COMPLEX SYSTEMS

Fritjof Capra's (2002) work on complex systems identifies three intertwined aspects of a system:

1. *Structures:* the concrete attributes or features of the system
2. *Processes:* the sequences of events
3. *Patterns:* phenomena and behaviors

Bringing about complex organizational change requires an understanding of the interactions among these three elements. Traditional or "classic" improvement work has focused mainly on changes in the structures and processes of a complex system, while patterns have been left largely unaltered. The natural next step in the evolution of improvement methods is to shed light on this third element.

FIVE KEY PATTERNS

While many patterns of behavior and phenomena exist in a system that is as complex as a typical healthcare organization, the following five patterns often have the greatest effect on the ability of an organization to change:

1. The nature of relationships
2. How decisions are made
3. How power is defined, acquired, and used
4. How conflict is handled
5. How learning is supported

Just as process mapping (or flowcharting) is about explicitly identifying the current and desired flow of people, information, and materials in a complex system, *pattern mapping* is about explicitly identifying the current and desired patterns in these five key dimensions. The method for mapping involves creating rich and honest conversation around a set of provocative questions related to each dimension. This dialog is essential to understanding how these patterns positively and negatively affect the thinking and actions that may facilitate or hinder transformational change.

The key question related to the "relationships" pattern (#1) is, Do the interactions among the various parts of the system generate energy and innovative ideas for change, or do they drain the organization? Examples of relationship patterns that have emerged in dialog among organizational leaders in healthcare include the following:

- The only time we ever talk is when there is a problem or issue—we do not really take much time out for relationship building.
- Relationships are very much shaped by the personalities of the senior leaders.

Determining whether, and to what extent, these patterns are energy generating or energy draining requires further investigation and discussion, but asking the question is the crucial first step.

The key question related to the "decision making" pattern (#2) is, Are decisions about change made rapidly and by the people with the most knowledge of the issue, or is change bogged down in hierarchy and position authority? Some examples of decision making patterns are as follows:

- Decisions are made pretty quickly, with lots of opportunity for everyone to provide input.
- Clinicians rarely get a chance to give input in decision making on managerial issues.
- Committee representatives are not empowered to make decisions and must take everything back to their departments for discussion, which makes decision making on even simple things very slow.

The key question related to the "power" pattern (#3) is, Do individuals and groups acquire and exercise power in positive, constructive ways toward a collective purpose, or is power coveted and used mainly for self-interest and self-preservation? Some examples of power patterns include the following:

- While power is generally exercised in a wonderful, open, inclusive, and constructive manner, there is sometimes frustration about all the talking and how much time it takes to make even simple decisions.
- Power is generally acquired and used in traditional ways; that is, formal senior leaders have the power to allocate budgets, hold others accountable, and so on.

Whether you think power is being used constructively depends on whether you happen to agree with the point of view taken by the powerful few. If you do not agree, there is little you can do about it; individuals without position-power have little voice in the system.

The key question related to the "conflict" pattern (#4) is, Are conflicts and differences of opinion embraced as opportunities to discover new ways of working, or are these seen as negative and destructive? Some examples of conflict patterns are listed below:

- We tend to avoid conflict. We say, "Let's take the heat out of this," but that also takes the energy out of things and we go nowhere.
- Conflict is completely underground around here. Everyone is expected to act very nice and polite and to behave as though they are totally on board with whatever the organization is saying. Other viewpoints are expressed only in private conversations. This leads to lots of talk about supporting change, but actually very little change.

The key question related to the "learning" pattern (#5) is, Is the system naturally curious and eager to learn more about itself and about what might be better, or is new thinking viewed mainly as potentially risky and threatening to the status quo? Some examples of learning patterns include the following:

- We learn well from outside experts; we are keen to try out new ideas and approaches. What we do less well is learning from our own people who often have very good ideas and lots to contribute.
- We are so task- and target-driven that we rarely take the time to stop and reflect on what we are doing or learning.

FACILITATING PATTERN MAPPING

Initiating and capturing the dialog generated from these questions obviously require good facilitation skills, but quality improvement team facilitators usually have the necessary skills to do so. What is needed is the application of those facilitation skills beyond discussions about processes to enable us to talk about the patterns that exist in our systems.

In a typical pattern mapping session, a group of leaders, clinicians, and staff assemble around a specific issue or subsystem. For example, a group may want to map patterns associated with emergency services, the new cancer care center, the corporate leadership team, or the coordination of care for elderly patients in a community. Having a specific focus grounds the conversation in reality and enables specific actions to make things better following the dialog.

Small group discussions with 5 to 12 people at a table provide a good mix of opinions and the opportunity for everyone to speak. The facilitator (or team of facilitators, if the group is large) introduces the provocative questions and asks the group to describe the current patterns first and then the desired patterns next to achieve the transformation or improvement goals of the system. Drawing a vertical line down the center of a piece of flipchart paper and labeling the left column "Current Patterns" and the other "Desired Patterns" creates a nice visual contrast between what exists now and what the group knows they need. A common response on evaluation sheets at the end of such a session is, "We have never had a conversation like this before, but we really needed it!"

Typically, groups need about 45 to 60 minutes of discussion to fully explore each pattern. It is not strictly necessary to cover all five patterns, and different groups can work on different patterns and then share results.

The next key step involves synthesizing the information and action planning. Pioneering work on pattern mapping with groups in the National Health Service (NHS) in the United Kingdom indicates that this step is best done in follow-up sessions, allowing for some time to pass and for personal reflection to occur after the intensity of the initial dialog. Synthesizing and action planning involve seeing the linkages between the various structures, processes, and patterns in the system and testing changes (for example, using PDSA cycles) to alter the system in more productive directions that will enable transformation. The linkages can be shown on a relationship diagram, like the one shown in Figure I, where all of the flipchart sheets from the five patterns are displayed on a large wall and a string or tape is used to indicate how each current and desired pattern relates to others. Symbols can be used to indicate whether the relationship is reinforcing (+) or hindering (–).

For example, we may observe that our structure of cross-departmental committees is hindering our transformation efforts because the pattern of having departmental representatives who do not have the power to make decisions results in very slow decision making. Further, we may notice that we have a pattern of unintended conflict and slow learning because our internal process for sharing information is not very good. Therefore, an action plan may involve reexamining the committee charters to say that

Figure I. Pattern Map

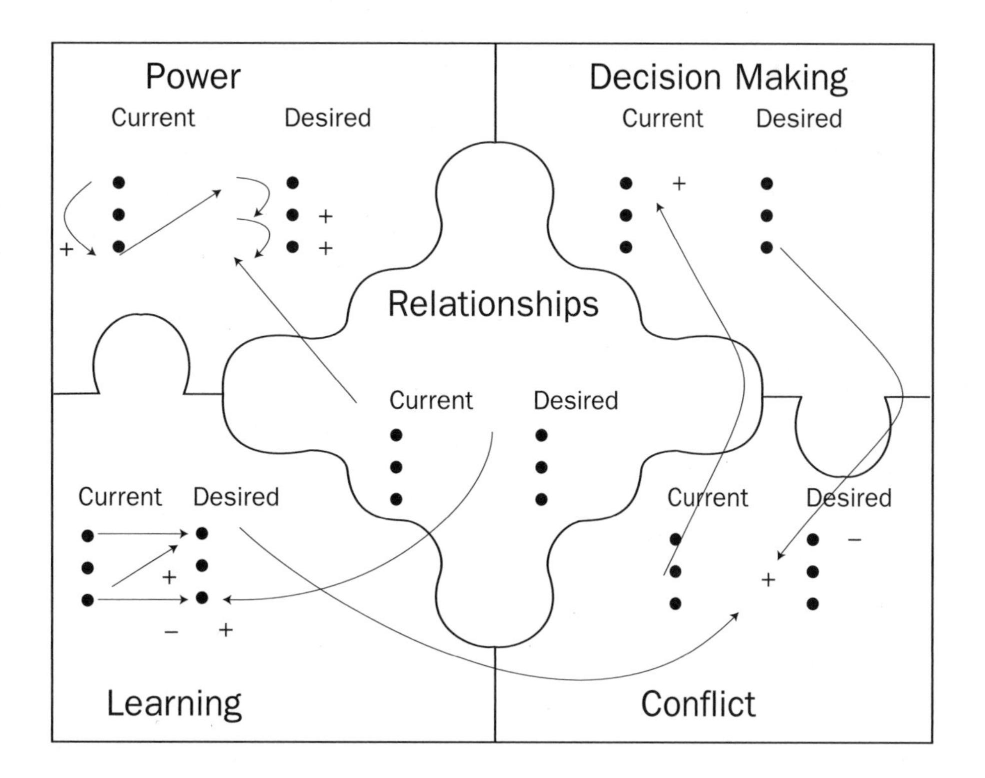

departmental representatives are fully empowered to make decisions for their departments; or we might try a committee meeting process that gives everyone ten minutes to call back to their departments in the middle of the meeting to immediately identify any issues or get approval on a decision so that the matter can be closed then and there.

EXAMPLE: NHS OPHTHALMOLOGY SERVICE

The ophthalmology service in a large hospital in England was described by organizational leaders as being "in crisis." The service was way behind in meeting its performance targets; other departments had a very low opinion of them; there was little sense of teamwork; constant friction between clinicians and management existed; and, despite the best efforts of improvement advisors, little progress was being made in improving the system. Something new was needed to unblock the situation.

Leaders asked for help from the NHS Modernisation Agency's Pursuing Perfection Team. They set up a workshop for all staff, including clinicians, managers, clerical staff, and some external stakeholders. They established a new way of thinking by setting improvement goals in the form of "promises to patients," rather than as performance targets. Then they began exploring whether the structures, processes, and patterns in the service were capable of delivering on those promises. The need to focus on the patterns of relationships between managers and clinicians emerged as the key issue that was clearly impeding any transformation of the service. The group engaged in some deeply honest (and, at times, difficult) dialog about this and mapped the current and desired patterns of relationships. As noted in the quote at the beginning of this chapter, this was like "letting the genie out of the bottle."

The staff in the service discussed many long-term frustrations and feelings of disempowerment. The CEO accepted the feedback and committed to take action on key issues, while the staff finally felt listened to and empowered to make change. Structure and process changes that emerged from the pattern mapping included new management located on-site within the service (previously, the manager had split responsibilities for, and was physically located within,

Figure J. Example of Improvement in a Key Indicator After Pattern Mapping

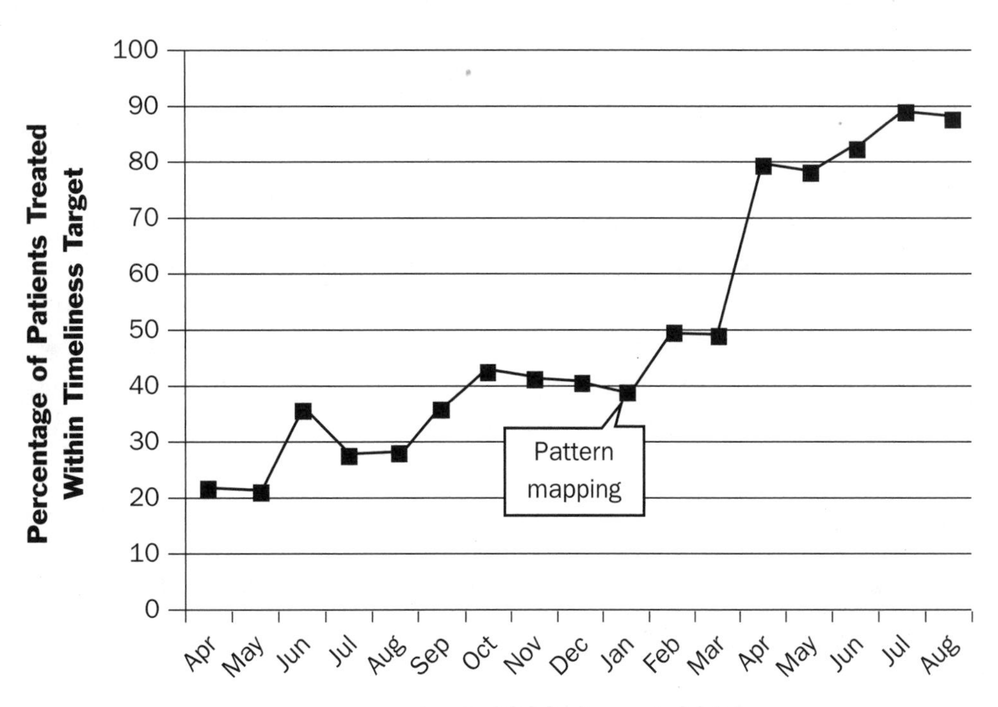

another service) and redesigned care pathways to improve flow and efficiency. Examples of changes in patterns included the following:

- From difficulty getting staff to work to staff calling in on their day off to offer help to achieve the department's targets
- From staff bringing problems and complaints to managers to fix to staff saying, "this was the problem, and this is what we have already done about it"
- From senior leaders thinking that clinicians were only interested in lining their pockets to clinicians delivering on their promises to patients.

Figure J illustrates the dramatic improvement in performance on a key indicator that occurred after the pattern-mapping event.

Sunlight is said to be among the best disinfectants. Too often, large organizations are infected by patterns of behavior and phenomena that impede positive progress toward systemwide improvement. Simultaneously, patterns exist—especially in organizations devoted to, and experienced in, improvement work—that can facilitate and accelerate large-scale improvement efforts. However, these positive patterns, just like the negative ones, often exist unnoticed. Pattern mapping is a promising, next-generation tool for any organizational improvement effort.

WHERE TO LEARN MORE

Sarah Garrett and Jo Bibby (formerly of the NHS Modernisation Agency) were codevelopers, along with Paul Plsek, of the concept and tools for pattern mapping. For more information about pattern mapping and its application in the National Health Service in the United Kingdom, please read the following documents online:

- http://www.directedcreativity.com/pages/PatternsOnePage.pdf.
- http://www.directedcreativity.com/pages/PatternMapping(final).pdf.
- http://www.directedcreativity.com/pages/PatternMapPoster.pdf.
- http://www.modern.nhs.uk/scripts/default.asp?site_id=40&id=24698.

REFERENCE

Capra, F. 2002. *The Hidden Connections: Integrating the Biological, Cognitive, and Social Dimensions of Life into a Science of Sustainability*. New York: Doubleday.

IDEA 5

Implement Rapid Response Teams

"... if we are to improve the quality of the decisions we make, we need to accept the mysterious nature of our snap judgments. We need to respect the fact that it is possible to know without knowing why we know and accept that—sometimes—we're better off that way."

—Malcolm Gladwell, *Blink*

Of all the ideas presented in this book, perhaps no other has the life-saving potential of rapid response teams. Research shows that the majority of critical inpatient events are preceded by warning signs for an average of six hours (Franklin and Matthew 1994). Rapid response teams (RRTs), also referred to as medical emergency teams, rescue patients in trouble and intervene before critical or lethal problems develop. An RRT is a small but powerful team experienced at assessing patient symptoms and conditions. It is a team continuously and readily available to respond to any provider who wants a second opinion about a patient who is showing signs of decline. Although some ▸

studies question whether the use of RRTs significantly reduces the incidence of cardiac arrest or unexpected death, other studies show up to a 50 percent reduction in non-ICU cardiac arrests (Hillman et al. 2005; Buist et al. 2002).

WHY RAPID RESPONSE TEAMS?

The need for a team specifically formed and designed to respond to patients whose condition is deteriorating stems from three fundamental problems within the care setting:

1. Failures in planning (including assessments, treatments, and goals)
2. Failure to communicate (patient-to-staff, staff-to-staff, staff-to-physician)
3. Failure to recognize deteriorating patient condition

These three problems, when left unaddressed, can often lead to a lethal failure: the *failure to rescue* a critical patient.

ACTING ON INSTINCT

One of the key elements of this emerging approach is *empowerment*. Having an RRT in place empowers caregivers to act quickly and effectively, even when an assessment or diagnosis is not clear. Too often, staff members feel reluctant to act on instinct or gut feeling. This reluctance sometimes stems from an inability to clearly articulate what the staff member observes as signs of trouble or decline. A call to the patient's doctor or to the doctor on call can prove fruitless if the information provided does not properly alert the doctor to a developing problem. An RRT eliminates this communication gap. A gut feeling triggers a call to the RRT, which allows for a more comprehensive assessment of the patient's condition. This assessment, performed by a team focused on looking for early signs of deterioration, can then lead to life-saving treatment.

For those who may be skeptical of placing such importance on instinct or gut feeling, consider Malcolm Gladwell's (2005) assertion that a gut feeling is the result of real, analytical reasoning that occurs in one's unconscious. In *Blink*, Gladwell writes, " ... if we are to improve the quality of the decisions we make, we need to accept the mysterious nature of our snap judgments. We need to respect the fact that it is possible to know without knowing why we know and accept that—sometimes—we're better off that way."

Respecting this " ... know[ing] without knowing why we know ... " is critical if a healthcare professional senses danger without being able to articulate, or even know, *why* he or she senses it. The reluctance to call an RRT because of this inability to articulate or understand a gut feeling needs to be overcome if RRTs are to fulfill their promise.

Several scientific studies tell us that most patients deteriorate for hours before cardiac arrest and have clearly identifiable warning signs (Schein 1990; Franklin and Matthew 1994). At the same time, studies of organizational behavior and management tell us that new, inexperienced staff are often unsure about when to call for help. This is a case in which science and "the gut" have the potential to work together for improved patient safety.

DESIGN AND IMPLEMENTATION OF AN RRT

When designing and implementing RRTs, the following steps should be taken:

- Engage senior leadership support.
- Determine the best structure for the team.
- Provide education and training.
- Establish criteria and a mechanism for calling the RRT.
- Use a structured documentation tool.
- Establish feedback mechanisms.
- Measure effectiveness of the RRT and improve the processes over time.

Engage senior leadership support. As with any improvement effort, the support of senior leadership—both physicians and executives—is essential. Perhaps the most important task for senior leaders is the development of a clear and broad communication strategy. First and most important, senior leaders signal the organization's explicit commitment to establishing the RRT; their message to the organization must be loud and clear: We are going to do this; this is important and the right thing to do for our patients. In addition, senior leaders must educate the medical staff about the benefits of an RRT and put the myths to rest. A potential barrier faced by senior leaders is the perception, often by physicians, that the status quo is both simple and sufficient (e.g., "The nurse calls, and I respond."). The reality is that communication challenges—for example, a new nurse, unsure of his or her assessment of the patient's condition, trying to communicate that assessment to a busy physician in a busy setting—can be dangerous. It is important for senior leaders to design and implement a plan with a willing team, work out the issues and problems, and then spread the RRT model across the entire organization. Another challenge for leaders is to create a reward system for calling for help to overcome reluctance on the part of nurses, especially those who are new or less experienced, to call the RRT.

Determine the best structure for the team. When determining the structure and make-up of the RRT, three considerations are paramount: (1) availability of both staff and resources, (2) accessibility (team members must have access to the patient and to the relevant patient information), and (3) ability (team members must have the experience and confidence to act quickly). While there is no set composition of an RRT, consider the following models:

1. An ICU registered nurse (RN) and respiratory therapist (RT)
2. An ICU RN, RT, intensivist, and resident
3. An ICU RN, RT, and intensivist or hospitalist
4. An ICU RN, RT, and physician assistant

Do you notice the common elements in these models? A nurse experienced and trained in an ICU is essential to any effective RRT. Because difficulty breathing is so often a sign of a developing or potential problem, a respiratory therapist is enormously valuable to the team. These models are not meant to be prescriptive, but they should provide guidelines for the selection of an appropriate team.

Provide education and training. Educating and training staff—all staff, not just members of the RRT—is essential to the effectiveness of an RRT. In addition to specific training, all medical staff should be educated about the benefits of these teams. RRT members themselves need to be educated and trained in advanced cardiac life support or other types of advanced critical care. They should be familiar with the SBAR (Situation, Background, Assessment, Recommendation) method of communication (see Idea 10). They need to understand the importance of clinical prediction and timely response. Finally, they need to understand the importance of providing nonjudgmental, supportive feedback to the call initiator. Because nurses are most likely to initiate the call, the nursing staff in general needs to clearly understand or have a mastery of (1) the criteria for calling the RRT, (2) the notification process, and (3) the necessary communication and teamwork skills.

Establish criteria and a mechanism for calling the RRT. Establishing the criteria for calling the RRT is of critical importance. Note that these are only suggestions; the very idea of establishing a rigid criteria list works against one of the most important aspects of the RRT idea—namely the need for staff members to feel comfortable calling the RRT *even when unsure of the exact nature of the problem.* That said, these criteria have been used effectively by some of the teams that have implemented RRTs:

- Staff member is worried about the patient
- Acute change in heart rate < 40 or > 130 bpm
- Acute change in systolic blood pressure < 90 mmHg
- Acute change in respiratory rate < 8 or > 28 per minute
- Acute change in saturation < 90 percent despite oxygen
- Acute change in conscious state
- Acute change in urinary output to < 50 ml in 4 hours

Establishing the mechanism for calling the RRT is of obvious importance. The mechanism should be clearly and widely understood by all staff members. Call initiators should be encouraged to dial from the patient's room. If not in the patient room, the call initiator should clearly communicate the location of the patient to the RRT.

Use a structured documentation tool, and *establish feedback mechanisms.* All the data from the RRT call, from the reason for the call to the specific intervention undertaken, should be documented. The data can then be used to assess and improve the design of the team and its processes. Associated with this need for structured documentation is the need for feedback mechanisms. A structured process should be in place for providing feedback regarding the patient outcome and any questions or problems noticed by staff members. This feedback should be used to design and drive future educational programs.

Figure K. Baptist Memorial Hospital: Percentage of Coded Patients Surviving at Discharge

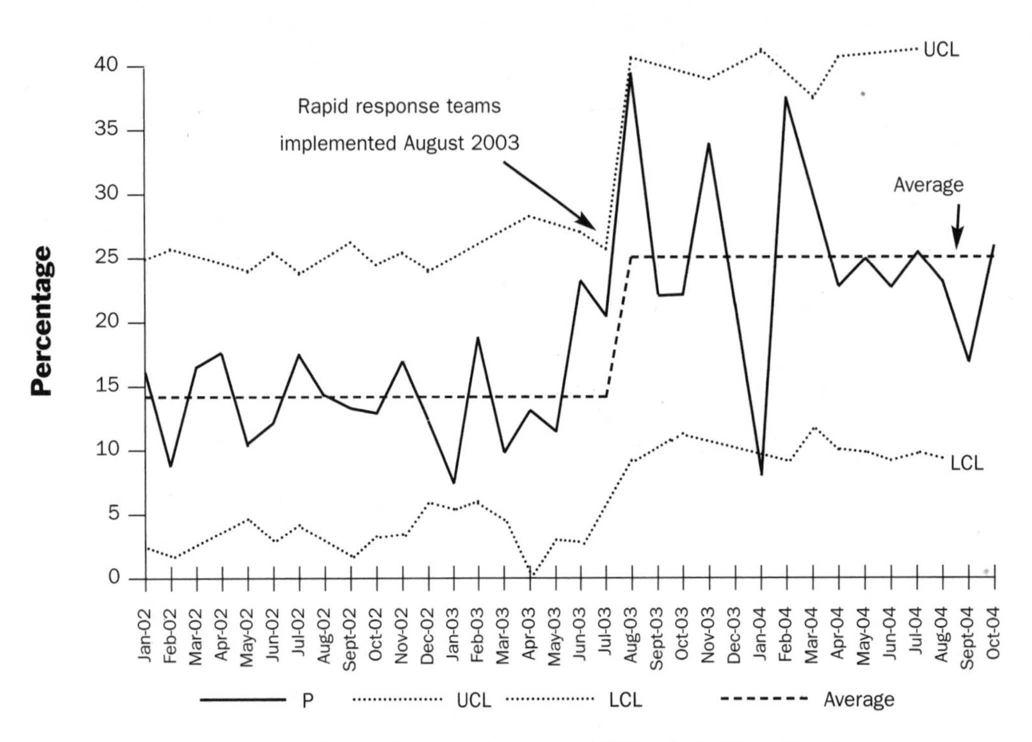

Source: Reprinted with permission from Baptist Memorial Hospital, Memphis, Tennessee.

Remember, share the success stories! Disseminating these stories is essential to building confidence in the RRT.

Measure effectiveness of the RRT. Careful measurement should be employed to study the effectiveness of the RRT and to identify areas where improvement is needed. When designing a measurement process, consider the following measures:

- Codes per 1,000 discharges
- Percent of codes outside the ICU
- Number of RRT calls
- Percent of coded patients surviving at discharge

EXAMPLE: BAPTIST MEMORIAL HOSPITAL

As part of an overall effort to reduce hospital mortality, Baptist Memorial Hospital in Memphis, Tennessee,

Figure L. Baptist Memorial Hospital: Percentage of Hospital Codes per 1,000 Discharges

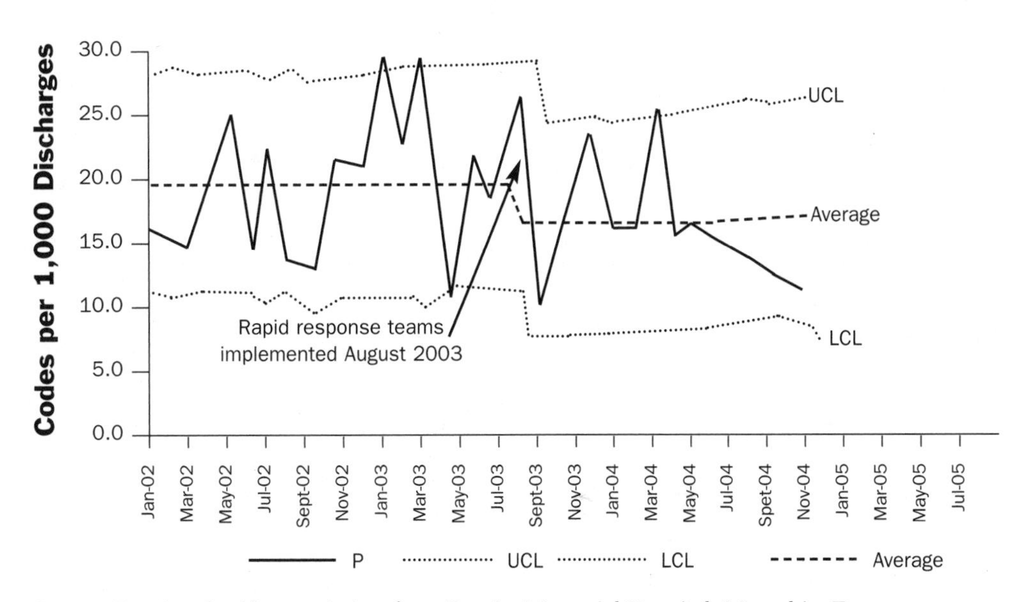

Source: Reprinted with permission from Baptist Memorial Hospital, Memphis, Tennessee.

implemented what it refers to as "Medical Response Teams." The design and structure of the medical response teams (MRTs) follows many of the suggestions and guidelines detailed in this chapter. At Baptist Memorial, any staff member can initiate a consult. The hospital developed the following "trigger" list that prompts any staff member to alert the MRT:

- A staff member is worried about a patient.
- There is an acute change in heart rate.
- There is an acute change in systolic blood pressure.
- There is an acute change in respiratory rate.
- There is an acute change in oxygen saturation.
- There is an acute change in level of consciousness.

The team at Baptist Memorial found that an average of 21 calls were made to their MRT per week. The results were impressive:

- The percent of coded patients surviving at discharge increased from an average of just under 15 percent before MRTs were implemented to approximately 25 percent afterward (see Figure K on page 40).
- Codes per 1,000 discharges decreased from an average of approximately 20 to an average of approximately 15 (see Figure L on page 41).

WHERE TO LEARN MORE

Bristow, P. J., K. M. Hillman, T. Chey, K. Daffurn, T. C. Jacques, S. L. Norman, G. F. Bishop, and E. G. Simmons. 2000. "Rates of In-Hospital Arrests, Deaths, and Intensive Care Admissions: The Effect of a Medical Emergency Team." *Medical Journal of Australia* 173 (5): 236–40.

"Improvement Story: Rapid Response Teams: Heading Off Medical Crises at Baptist Memorial Hospital-Memphis." See the story on http://www.ihi.org/IHI/Topics/Improvement/MoveYourDot/ImprovementStories/RapidResponseTeamsHeadingOffMedicalCrisesatBaptistMemorialHospitalinMemphis.htm.

For more information on implementing RRTs as part of IHI's *100,000 Lives Campaign*, please visit http://www.ihi.org/IHI/Programs/Campaign/Campaign.htm?TabId=2#Deploy%20Rapid%20Response%20Teams.

REFERENCES

Buist, M. D., G. E. Moore, S. A. Bernard, B. P. Waxman, J. N. Anderson, and T. V. Nguyen. 2002. "Effects of a Medical Emergency Team on Reduction of Incidence of and Mortality from Unexpected Cardiac Arrests in Hospital: Preliminary Study." *British Medical Journal* 324 (7334): 387–90.

Franklin, C., and J. Mathew. 1994. "Developing Strategies to Prevent Inhospital Cardiac Arrest: Analyzing Responses of Physicians and Nurses in the Hours Before the Event." *Critical Care Medicine* 22 (2): 244–47.

Gladwell, M. 2005. *Blink*. New York: Little Brown and Company.

Hillman, K., J. Chen, M. Cretikos, R. Bellomo, D. Brown, G. Doig, S. Finfer, A. Flabouris, and MERIT study investigators. 2005. "Introduction of the Medical Emergency Team (MET) System: A Cluster-Randomised Controlled Trial." *Lancet* 365 (9477): 2091–97.

Schein, R. M., N. Hazday, M. Pena, B. H. Ruben, and C. L. Sprung. 1990. "Clinical Antecedents to In-Hospital Cardiopulmonary Arrest." *Chest* 98 (6) 1388–92.

IDEA 6

Reconcile Medications at Every Handoff

"To err is human, but errors can be prevented."
—*To Err Is Human: Building a Safer Health System* (Institute of Medicine)

Of all the things that can go wrong during a hospital stay, few are more frightening than a medication error. Drugs that are designed to treat, heal, and cure can become lethal if administered wrongly. Injuries that result from a wrongly administered medication are known as adverse drug events (ADEs). A patient who experiences an ADE is almost twice as likely to die as a patient who does not (Classen et al. 1997). In 1993, according to data culled from death certificates, medication errors led to approximately 1,200 in-hospital deaths (Phillips, Christenfeld, and Glynn 1998). With the healthcare world flooded with more and more medications, it is not surprising that the rate of lethal ADEs more than doubled in the period between 1983 and 1993 ▸

(Phillips, Christenfeld, and Glynn 1998).

The problem continues to grow: The Institute of Medicine (IOM) report, *To Err Is Human*, estimates that more than 7,000 deaths per year are caused by medication errors (Kohn, Corrigan, and Donaldson 1999). Predictably, these errors are also a financial drain on the industry. ADEs account for 6.3 percent of malpractice suits (Rothschild et al. 2002). Both the IOM and the Joint Commission on Accreditation of Healthcare Organizations have identified the prevention of ADEs as a national priority.

Several methods of preventing ADEs exist, but this chapter focuses on a method that targets the most dangerous point in a patient's path through a hospital stay: the transition from one care location to another. At these "handoffs" is where errors often occur. The solution we propose is *medication reconciliation at every handoff*. Medications not reconciled at all transition points may account for up to 46 percent of medication errors and 20 percent of ADEs (Pronovost et al. 2003; Rozich and Resar 2001). Medication reconciliation ensures that patients receive nothing but the intended medications following a transition to another care location. Medication reconciliation is the process of creating the most accurate list possible of all medications that a patient is taking and comparing that list against the physician's admission, transfer, or discharge orders. This list should include the drug name, dosage, frequency, and route.

The goal of this idea is to provide correct medications to the patient at all transition points within the hospital or between other care sites (e.g., between the ICU and medical floors, from the hospital to the home).

TIPS FOR AVOIDING ERRORS AT TRANSITION POINTS

The suggestions below are by no means exhaustive, but they should compel leaders to identify the areas within the healthcare setting where problems are likely to occur.

1. Develop policies to ensure that when a patient is transferred out of the ICU, medications that are not appropriate for the next setting are discontinued automatically.
2. Create a standardized form that lists all the medications the patient was taking at home (prior to admission) and that the physician

can use as an order form. Include space for the physician to document reasons for omitting medications.
3. Follow the same reconciliation procedure for surgical patients. Compare the preoperative medication orders to the postoperative medications, and reconcile any discrepancies.

EXAMPLE: LUTHER MIDELFORT HOSPITAL

Consider the case of Luther Midelfort Hospital (part of the Mayo Health System) in Eau Claire, Wisconsin. The team formed to reduce actual and potential ADEs reviewed patient records and found that up to 50 percent of all medication errors and up to 20 percent of ADEs (both in the hospital and in outpatient settings) were attributable to medications not reconciled at transition points. Compelled by this troubling discovery, the team took the following steps to address the problem:

1. Developed a tool called the "Medication Reconciliation Data Collection Form" (see Figure M) for reconciling medications at admission, identifying discrepancies, and capturing documentation. This form reduces the need for nurses and pharmacists to contact physicians for clarification.
2. Redesigned the discharge process, using new forms that required a review for reconciliation of medications. This step ensures that patients left the hospital with accurate discharge instructions and medication orders.
3. Required a reconciliation review of each patient's medication administration record (MAR) during transfer between patient care units. This review ensures that medications are not inadvertently omitted.
4. Recruited a team to redesign (i.e., error-proof) the MAR.
5. Established a quality audit of the reconciliation review process and data-reporting procedures.
6. Started performing medication reconciliation during admissions to the critical care unit.

The results were extremely encouraging. Figure N (on page 47) shows the errors on reviewed charts per 100 admissions (the Y-axis) plotted against the six-month time period (the X-axis), during which medication reconciliation was initiated at various points in the care

Figure M. Luther Midelfort Hospital: Medication Reconciliation Data Collection Form

Errors from Unreconciled Medications

Patient Record	Review Date	Errors at Admission	Errors During Transfer	Errors at Discharge	Total Errors	Number of Records Reviewed
1						
2						
3						
4						
5						
Etc.						
					Total Errors from Records Reviewed	Total Records Reviewed

Source: Reprinted with permission from Luther Midelfort Hospital, Mayo Health System, Eau Claire, Wisconsin.

process. Figure N clearly shows the powerful effect of reconciliation, in general, and the extremely compelling outcomes of reconciliation at each transition point, specifically. The Luther Midelfort team exceeded its initial goal of reducing ADEs and potential ADEs by 60 percent and

Figure N. Luther Midelfort Hospital: Errors per 100 Admissions During Medication Reconciliation Implementation

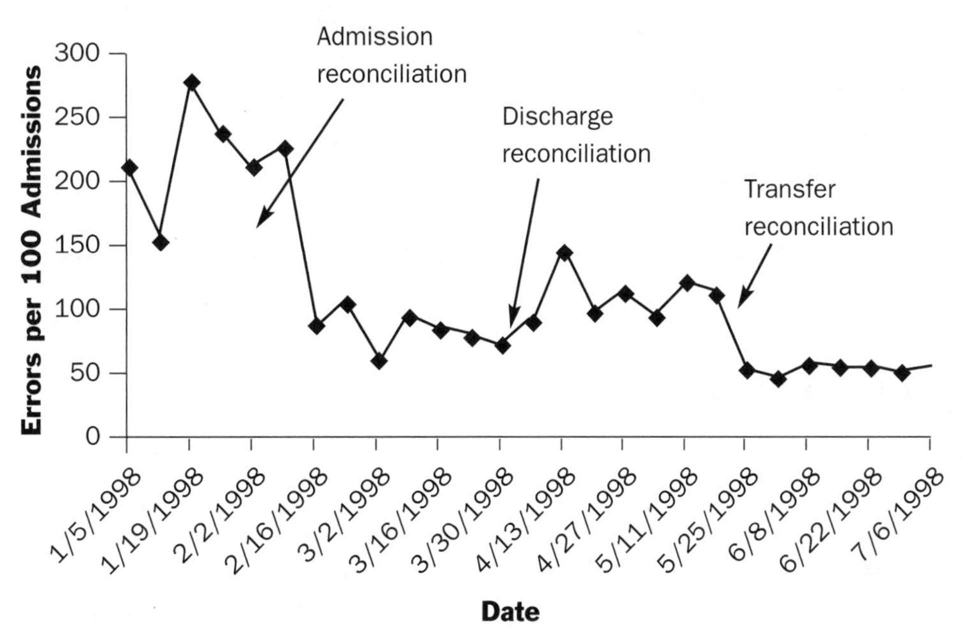

Source: Reprinted with permission from Luther Midelfort Hospital, Mayo Health System, Eau Claire, Wisconsin.

attributed this success in part to the implementation of reconciliation at admission, transfer, and discharge.

Now, six years after the team's early efforts, Luther Midelfort is holding the gains in reducing medication errors. These very encouraging results and their overall experience led the team to formulate the following four tips for implementing medication reconciliation:

1. Start with small, incremental tests of change. This is the best way to undertake a project of a large size.
2. Include all members of the patient care team in the process. No single group—nurses, pharmacists, or physicians—should be held responsible for ensuring that the process works.
3. Involve members of the staff and medical education departments early in the change process. They can help develop the tools to sustain the process with new staff and providers.
4. Measure and report the results.

This makes sustaining and expanding the improvement project possible.

The Joint Commission has studied the results at hospitals that have used medication reconciliation to drive down error rates and, as a result, now recommends that medication reconciliation be done at all handoffs.

WHERE TO LEARN MORE

For more information on JCAHO's 2005 Hospitals' National Patient Safety Goals, please visit http://www.jcaho.org/accredited+organizations/patient+safety/05+npsg/05_npsg_hap.htm

Medication reconciliation is one of six interventions included in IHI's 100,000 Lives Campaign. For more information, please visit http://www.ihi.org/IHI/Programs/Campaign/Campaign.htm?TabId=2#Prevent%20Adverse%20Drug%20Events.

The story of Luther Midelfort's experience can also be found on IHI's web site: http://www.ihi.org/IHI/Topics/PatientSafety/MedicationSystems/ImprovementStories/Reducing+ADEs+Through+Medication+Reconciliation.htm.

A similarly encouraging story of the effects of medication reconciliation from OSF Healthcare System in Peoria, Illinois, can be found on IHI's web site: http://www.ihi.org/IHI/Topics/PatientSafety/MedicationSystems/ImprovementStories/JourneyTowardsSafetyACulturalRevolution.htm.

REFERENCES

Classen, D. C., S. L. Pestotnik, R. S. Evans, J. F. Lloyd, and J. P. Burke. 1997. "Adverse Drug Events in Hospitalized Patients. Excess Length of Stay, Extra Costs, and Attributable Mortality." *JAMA* 277 (4): 301–06.

Kohn, L. T., J. M. Corrigan, and M. S. Donaldson (eds.). 1999. *To Err Is Human: Building a Safer Health System.* Washington, DC: National Academies Press, Institute of Medicine.

Phillips, D. P., N. Christenfeld, and L. M. Glynn. 1998. "Increase in U.S. Medication-Error Deaths Between 1983 and 1993." *Lancet* 351 (9103): 643–44.

Pronovost, P., B. Weast, M. Schwarz, R. M. Wyskiel, D. Prow, S. N. Milanovich, S. Berenholtz, T. Dorman, and P. Lipsett. 2003. "Medication Reconciliation: A Practical Tool to Reduce the Risk of Medication Errors." *Journal of Critical Care* 18 (4): 201–05.

Rothschild, J. M., F. A. Federico, T. K. Gandhi, R. Kaushal, D. H. Williams, and D. W. Bates. 2002. "Analysis of Medication-Related Malpractice Claims: Causes, Preventability, and Costs." *Archives of Internal Medicine* 162 (21): 2414–20.

Rozich, J. D., and R. K. Resar. 2001. "Medication Safety: One Organization's Approach to the Challenge." *Journal of Clinical Outcomes Management* 8 (10): 27–34.

IDEA 7

Develop Patient Itineraries

The goal is to be more predictive and less reactive.

This chapter is the first of three that deal with different aspects of patient flow. Patient itineraries are designed care paths that optimize sequence, distance, and value-added time for patients (and staff). It is a solution, and to understand it, a basic appreciation of the problem is essential.

OUTPATIENT FLOW: THE PROBLEM

Healthcare is organized around doctors' offices, outpatient surgery centers, rehabilitation centers, hospitals, pharmacies, and diagnostic centers. Because of this fragmented structure, patients must navigate a complex but suboptimized web of services. The following are key characteristics, and consequent problems, of that web:

- Care sites generally schedule appointments independently. Patients typically call one location for an appointment and, if referred to other locations for additional services, have to schedule those appointments separately. ▸

- Each care site makes little use of prediction of demand. Scheduling is then reactive, causing long patient queues to form.
- Lack of coordination between care sites results in redundant care processes.
- No care site looks at the capacity and demand of the entire system or manages the system's constraints.

These problems result in the following experiences.

For patients:

- Care that is uncoordinated, impersonal, and sometimes contradictory
- Delays in receiving the care they need and want, and when they need and want it
- Overly complex and inefficient systems that cause unnecessary delays and frustrations

For providers:

- Suboptimization—that is, providers have limited capacity to use their unique skills and expertise to do the work they are trained to do
- Actual or potential threats to financial viability
- A chaotic and stressful work life

THE PATIENT ITINERARY: A PROMISING SOLUTION

A patient itinerary can address many of these issues. By clearly specifying the necessary steps in the patient's care, the itinerary can maximize the value-added steps and minimize the non-value-added steps in the patient's care path. Every element of the care path should be considered as a step—for example, the wait time between initial suspicion of a problem and seeing a doctor is one step. This is a non-value-added step, however, and thus must be minimized.

Note that specifying each step does not mean that a patient itinerary is a rigidly defined sequence of steps. Whereas some steps in the patient care path are dependent on others, and thus part of a necessary sequence, other steps are not and thus can be scheduled in a manner that reduces waiting and increases the percentage of value-added time.

How does one create a patient itinerary? As with nearly everything in healthcare, this question has no one simple answer. When creating an itinerary, providers must use whatever information is available, be it in the form of a patient's history or the experience of a care provider. The goal is to be more predictive and less reactive. For example, a woman with a family or personal history of breast cancer who discovers a suspicious lump in a routine self-examination is likely to need an ultrasound in addition to a mammography. Realization of this need for diagnostic procedures *before* the woman arrives at the hospital or doctor's office to report her lump allows for advanced scheduling, reducing the patient's waiting time.

Another important consideration in creating an itinerary is demand versus capacity. If 20 women are scheduled to have ultrasounds on the same day, but the hospital has the capacity to perform only three per day, significant delays can result. Minimizing the difference between demand and capacity can greatly increase the efficiency of a care path.

The consistent thread between these different approaches is planning. At the core of patient itineraries is efficient planning, with the goal of maximizing value-added time. This goal is expressed in the following equation:

(Value-Added Time) ÷ (Total Cycle Time) > 20 percent

EXAMPLE: TWO SCENARIOS COMPARING VALUE-ADDED TIME

Consider the following two scenarios for breast cancer diagnosis—one represents a suboptimized flow path and the other a care path that uses a patient itinerary (see Figure O).

Scenario 1 represents the traditional patient journey. A patient calls for an appointment for diagnostic testing (mammogram and ultrasound). The appointment occurs four days after the call, and, as a result of the diagnostic tests, a biopsy is scheduled one week later. While the procedures themselves (value-added time) take only 2 hours, the entire cycle time (in business-day hours) is 74 hours. Thus, the percentage of value-added time within this week-long cycle is less than 5 percent.

Now look at Scenario 2. The same procedures are performed, and they take the same amount of time—two hours. By scheduling the original appointment two days after the initial call and the biopsy on the same day as the mammogram and ultrasound, the cycle time decreases from 74 hours to 19 hours. Note that, on occasion, the long cycle time in Scenario 1 is a matter of patient preference; some patients may want to wait a week before having the biopsy. In such

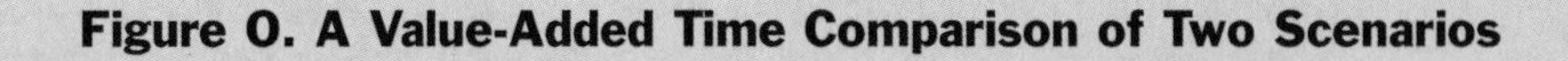
Figure O. A Value-Added Time Comparison of Two Scenarios

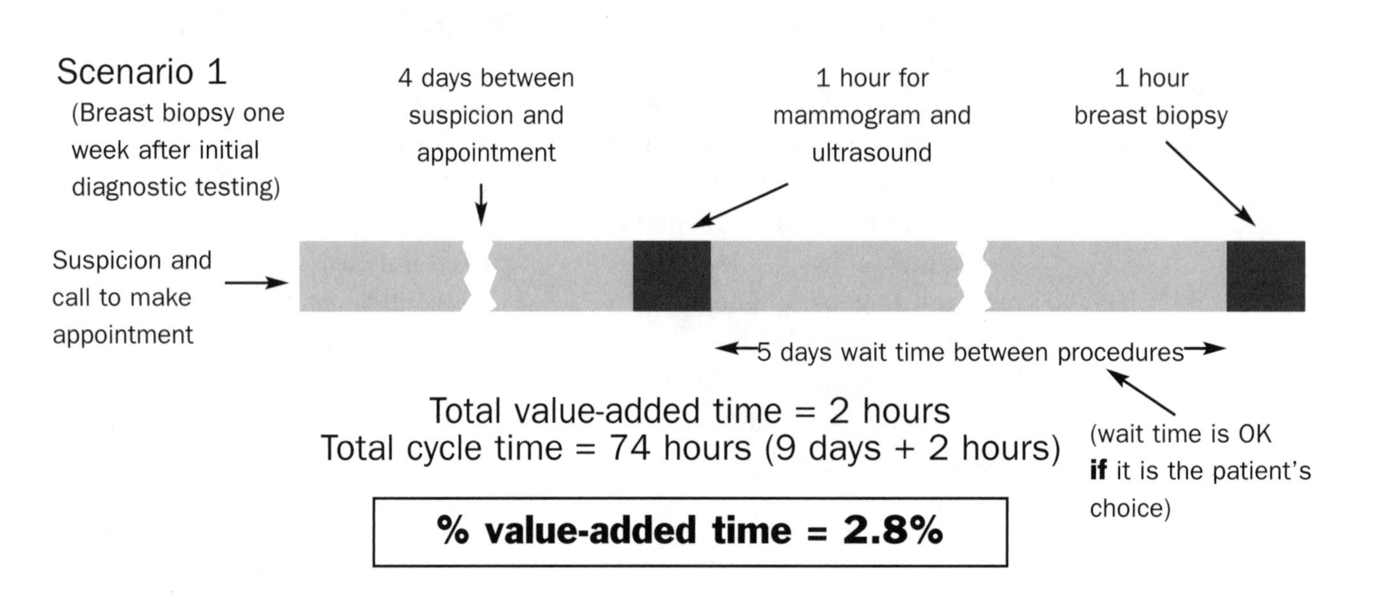
Scenario 1
(Breast biopsy one week after initial diagnostic testing)
4 days between suspicion and appointment
1 hour for mammogram and ultrasound
1 hour breast biopsy
Suspicion and call to make appointment
5 days wait time between procedures
Total value-added time = 2 hours
Total cycle time = 74 hours (9 days + 2 hours)
(wait time is OK if it is the patient's choice)
% value-added time = 2.8%

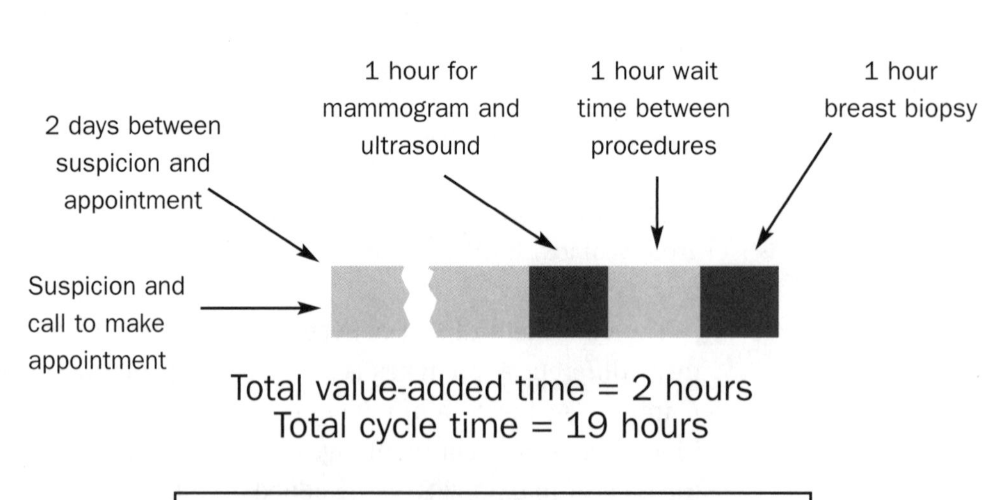
Scenario 2
(Breast biopsy same day as initial diagnostic testing)
2 days between suspicion and appointment
1 hour for mammogram and ultrasound
1 hour wait time between procedures
1 hour breast biopsy
Suspicion and call to make appointment
Total value-added time = 2 hours
Total cycle time = 19 hours
% value-added time = 10%

cases, it would be wrong to argue that the interim period is wholly without value. In most cases, however, patients want a complete diagnosis as soon as possible. Using a patient itinerary is a powerful way of optimizing the time it takes for a patient to get the necessary care.

Figure P. Steps in the Patient Care Path

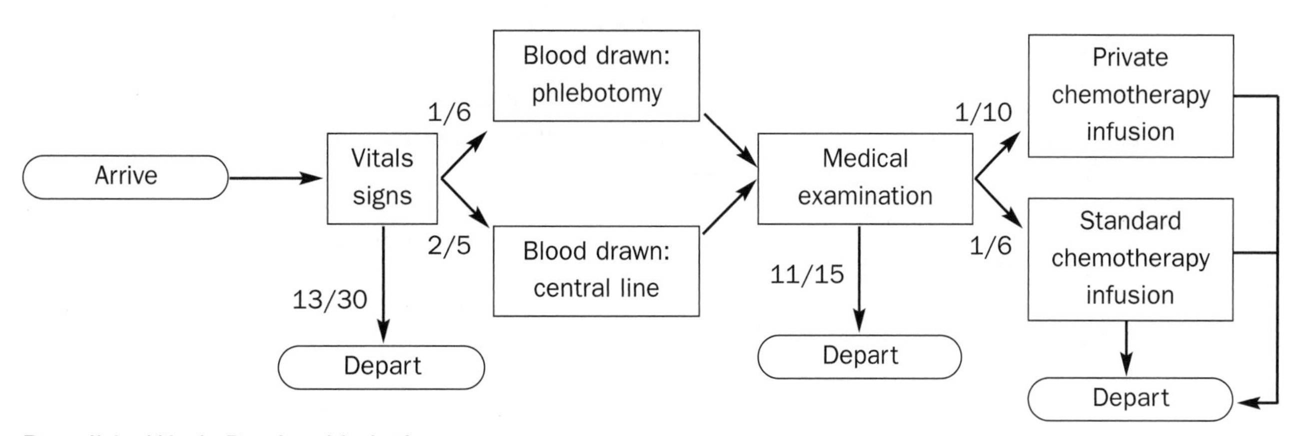

Possible Work Design Variations:

(Hard-wired sequencing)

1. Vitals → Draw blood → etc.
2. Draw blood → Vitals → etc.

(Adaptive, condition-based sequencing logic)

3. Get in shortest queue (Vitals or blood)
4. Do first available (Vitals or blood)

(Physical work design)

5. Services flow to patient, with all work in common room (motivation is shared resources = better throughput, flow, utilization)

Source: Reprinted with permission from Institute for Healthcare Improvement, Cambridge, Massachusetts.

EXAMPLE: REINIER DE GRAAF GASTHUIS

Reinier de Graaf Gasthuis, an academic medical center in Delft, the Netherlands, addressed its own flow problems in the breast care service area by redesigning the patient's journey from suspicion to diagnosis. By doing so, the hospital was able to reduce the typical number of visits, from two to three down to just one. The total cycle time was also reduced, from three to ten days to just three hours. The quality improvement team at Reinier de Graaf met to redesign care across the many sites that women had to navigate to get a diagnosis. The team reformed processes, handoffs, and communication to eliminate non-value-added time.

A team that seeks to get similar results achieved by Reinier de Graaf may map out the processes of care for a typical patient journey as a way to see new options. For example, the flow chart in Figure P (on page 55) shows normal steps in the course of patient care and the number of patients who take each route in the care path.

With input from the flow chart, the team can make the following improvements:

1. Design hard-wired sequences for patients with a predictable, often repetitive course of care.
2. Create flexible pathways for patients who need multiple services during a visit when the sequence of interactions does not need to follow a certain order.
3. Redesign the physical space to decrease travel time, waiting, and wasteful staff movement.

These design changes have been effective in many settings in driving down non-value-added time and can be combined with other flow and queuing tools. Providers focusing on the "white spaces" between process steps and on total cycle time, rather than looking at the work processes alone, is a paradigm shift.

WHERE TO LEARN MORE

For more information on patient flow, please visit IHI's web site: http://www.ihi.org/IHI/Topics/Flow.

IDEA 8

Measure Bed Turns and Test Changes to Improve Flow

Plot your dot.

Trends in the U.S. healthcare system show increases in hospital occupancy (percentage of beds that are filled) and in emergency department (ED) utilization. Bottlenecks, diversions, and cancellations then result, creating problems for patients and putting additional stress on staff. Innovations developed by IHI can offer hospitals new insights into their flow problems and a solution—measure hospital throughput and activity based on bed turns. A "bed turn" is defined as the number of times (rounded to the nearest whole number) a bed is used by a patient, whether for admission or for any type of observation. The goal of improving flow is fourfold:

1. increased throughput and minimized delays (more patients being moved through the hospital), ▸

2. decreased resource use (fewer beds being staffed and used for the same number of patients),
3. highest revenue per bed turn possible, and
4. maintained or improved level of quality of care.

THE HOSPITAL FLOW DIAGNOSTIC TOOL

The Hospital Flow Diagnostic Tool is a method for identifying areas of greatest need, based on bed turns and utilization, and then developing customized strategies for making changes to improve flow in those areas. (For a detailed explanation and instructions for use of the Hospital Flow Diagnostic Tool, please visit http://www.ihi.org/IHI/Topics/Flow/PatientFlow/EmergingContent/HospitalFlowDiagnostic.htm.)

Measuring bed turns as a way of understanding flow is a recent innovation, and testing is underway. By using this diagnostic tool, physicians, nurses, and staff gain a much better understanding of the flow problems in their own care setting.

The tool is a plot of adjusted bed turns versus utilization. The following formulas can help hospitals calculate their adjusted bed turns and utilization:

- Adjusted Bed Turns = [(Admissions × Case Mix Index) + Observations)]/Functional Beds
- Unadjusted Bed Turns = (Admissions + Observations)/Functional Beds
- Potential Bed Turns = 365 Days/Aggregate Length of Stay
- Utilization = Unadjusted Bed Turns/Potential Bed Turns

By plotting adjusted bed turns versus utilization, a hospital can determine in which quadrant of the tool it falls. Figure Q shows the results of plotting adjusted bed turns against utilization for several hospitals, each of which is represented by a single dot.

A hospital that falls into Quadrant 1 of the tool, with utilization of less than 90 and adjusted bed turns of greater than 90, efficiently matches beds and staffing with patient admissions; this is the "target quadrant" for hospitals that want to improve flow. A hospital that falls into Quadrant 2 has a higher number of admissions than available beds and staff, which results in overcrowding. A hospital that falls into Quadrant 3 often has more beds than patient admissions. A hospital that falls into Quadrant 4 often has a high average length of stay. The goal for hospitals that want to improve flow is to "move the dot" to Quadrant 1.

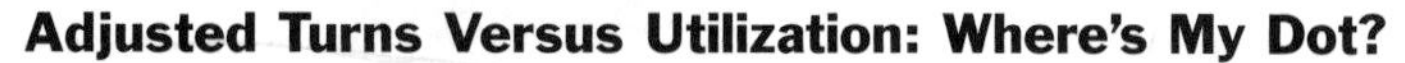

Figure Q. The Hospital Flow Diagnostic Tool

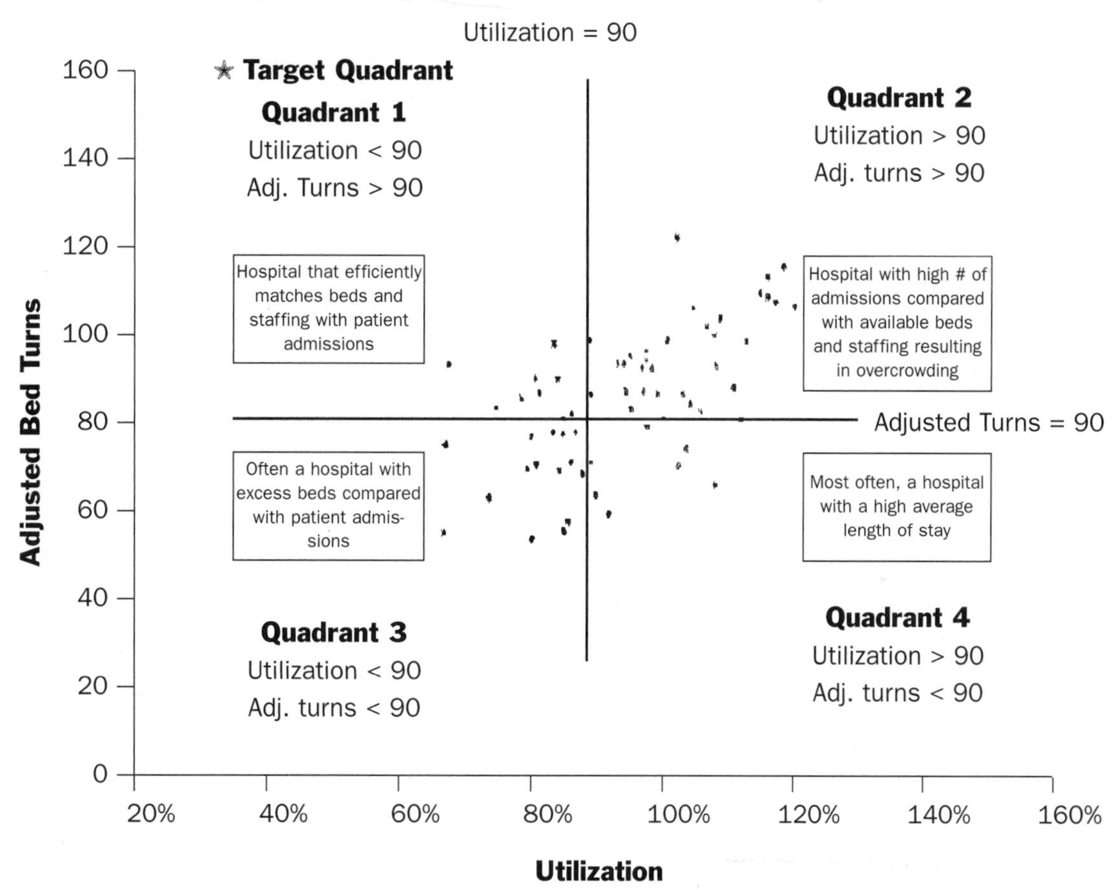

STRATEGIES FOR INCREASING THROUGHPUT

After using the tool to measure throughput and "plot your dot," a hospital will be able to identify the areas that are most in need of improvement. Below are some change concepts for addressing typical flow problem areas. Depending on which quadrant a hospital's dot falls into, the hospital can choose among a specific list of changes tailored to that quadrant.

Change concepts for eliminating delays (Quadrant 1):

- Reduce wasted slack capacity.
  - Eliminate bed holds.
  - Develop a room/bed cleaning and turnaround strategy.
  - Reduce internal transfers.
  - Decrease the use of inpatient beds by outpatients.
- Synchronize admissions, transfers, and discharges.
- Identify or remove bottlenecks.
- Add or shift capacity as needed.

Change concepts for decreasing length of stay (Quadrants 2 and 4):

- Use multidisciplinary rounds in units other than the ICU.
- Optimize staffing ratios.
- Focus on conditions that have a long length of stay compared to other hospitals.
- Predict and plan for admissions to extended care facilities.
- Conduct preadmission planning for elective surgery.
- Adhere to utilization criteria for specialty beds (e.g., telemetry, ICU, PACU).
- Reduce adverse events.

Change concepts for optimizing the use of existing capacity (Quadrant 2):

- Use discharge appointments and synchronize admissions, transfers, and discharges.
- Improve the capabilities of extended care facilities to preempt visits to the ED.
- Decrease readmissions.

Change concepts for increasing bed turns (Quadrants 3 and 4):

- Decrease variation in demand (e.g., smooth elective surgical admissions).
- Eliminate bed holds (e.g., holding a bed for a patient to be admitted after surgery).
- Develop a room/bed cleaning and turnaround strategy.
- Reduce internal transfers (consider acuity-adjustable beds—see Idea 9).
- Decrease use of inpatient beds by outpatients.
- Decrease capacity (e.g., convert semi-private to private rooms; do not staff to peaks in demand).

This is a long list of changes, far more than any single organization will implement. The point is to use the Hospital Flow Diagnostic Tool to understand your hospital's areas of greatest need and then to test changes that seem most promising for making improvements in those areas.

WHERE TO LEARN MORE

For more information on this topic, please visit IHI's web site: http://www.ihi.org/IHI/Topics/Flow/.

For additional information, please visit the Lean Enterprise Institute's web site: http://www.lean.org/.

IDEA 9

Adopt Acuity-Adjustable Beds and Rooms

The less a patient has to move around within a care setting, the better that patient's care will be.

The Center for Health Design, a research and advocacy group located in Concord, California, has collected evidence that shows that the physical design of a care setting can have profound effects on quality, safety, and patient satisfaction (Ulrich et al. 2004). Redesigning hospital environments can also improve staff retention. Noise, chaos, inconvenience, and reduced opportunities for direct patient care contribute to high nurse turnover. According to one observer, "We don't have a nursing shortage; we have a shortage of nurses willing to work in hospitals" (McCarthy 2004). One of these redesign efforts involves the building of acuity-adjustable beds and rooms.

One of the crucial flow problems experienced by hospital patients and staff is seen in the process of assigning critical-care and progressive-care beds and ▸

resources. On any given day, a large percentage of patients in these costly areas are misassigned and unable to move to an appropriate service because of downstream backlogs. Research shows that patients often move three to six times during a typical hospital stay to receive the care that matches their level of acuity (Hendrich, Fay, and Sorrells 2004). Each transfer is an opportunity for missed or delayed treatment, miscommunication that can lead to errors or omissions of care, patient falls, or other problems that are not only bad for patients but also consume additional staff time and resources.

BETTER DESIGN RESULTS IN BETTER OUTCOMES

A promising solution to this particular flow problem is acuity-adjustable beds. These beds, able to adapt to the patient's changing needs, represent improved care for patients as well as reductions in workload and stress on staff.

An extension of this idea is acuity-adjustable rooms, which are designed to make easily accessible all the equipment and supplies required for the medical needs of critical care patients. Headwalls can transform so that clinicians can administer advanced care. Computer technology is located directly on the patient's bed so that staff can record body weight and other vital data without disturbing the patient. Necessary supplies are in each patient's room, reducing "travel time" (excess motion) for nurses to and from a central supply location. Mini nursing stations, equipped with charts and computers, are located outside each patient room.

The effects of eliminating transfers are documented in a research study on the benefits of single rooms. This research (Hendrich, Fay, and Sorrells 2004) shows that single rooms are associated with the following results:

- Reduced nosocomial infections
- Reduced transfers and medical errors
- Less noise and stress for patients and staff
- Improved confidentiality and privacy
- Better social support by families
- Improved staff communications with patients
- Increased patient satisfaction

A central tenet of the work to improve patient flow is this: *The less a patient has to move around within a care setting, the better that patient's care (and thus outcome) will be.* Acuity-adjustable beds and rooms offer a promising solution to this problem of movement.

EXAMPLE: METHODIST HOSPITAL

The leadership at Methodist Hospital in Indianapolis, Indiana, decided to design and build 56 acuity-adjustable rooms. These acuity-adaptable units are designed to significantly reduce patient transfers by creating patient rooms that can accommodate low-risk and high-acuity patients.

The results were impressive:

- Transports from one level of acuity to another decreased by more than 90 percent (see Figure R)

Figure R. Methodist Hospital: Reduction in Transport of Patients Between UnitsUsing Acuity-Adaptable Rooms

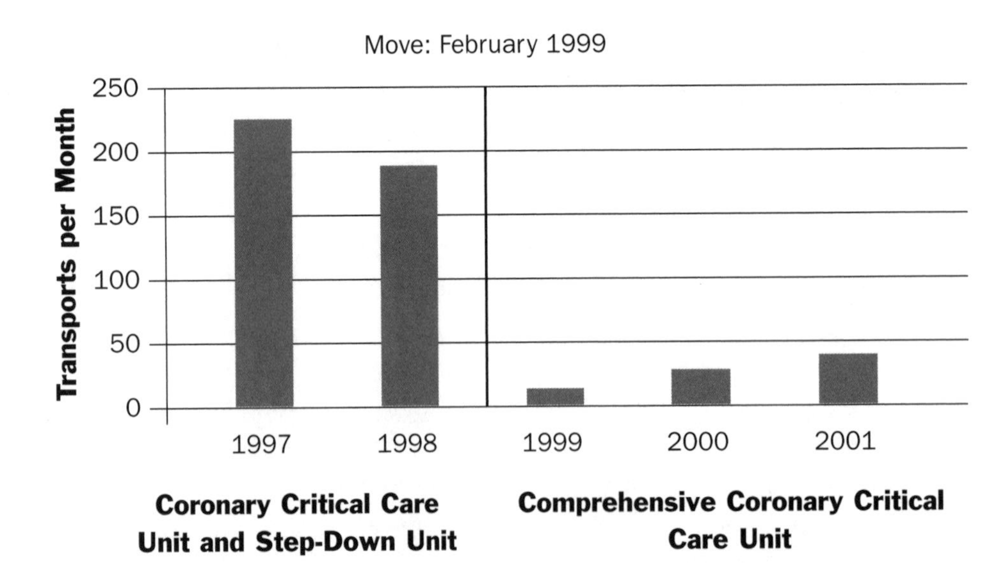

Source: Adapted from Hendrich, A., J. Fay, and A. K. Sorrells. 2004. "Effects of Acuity-Adaptable Rooms on Flow of Patients and Delivery of Care." *American Journal of Critical Care* 13 (1): 35–45.

Figure S. Methodist Hospital: Reduction in Annual Index for Medication Errors

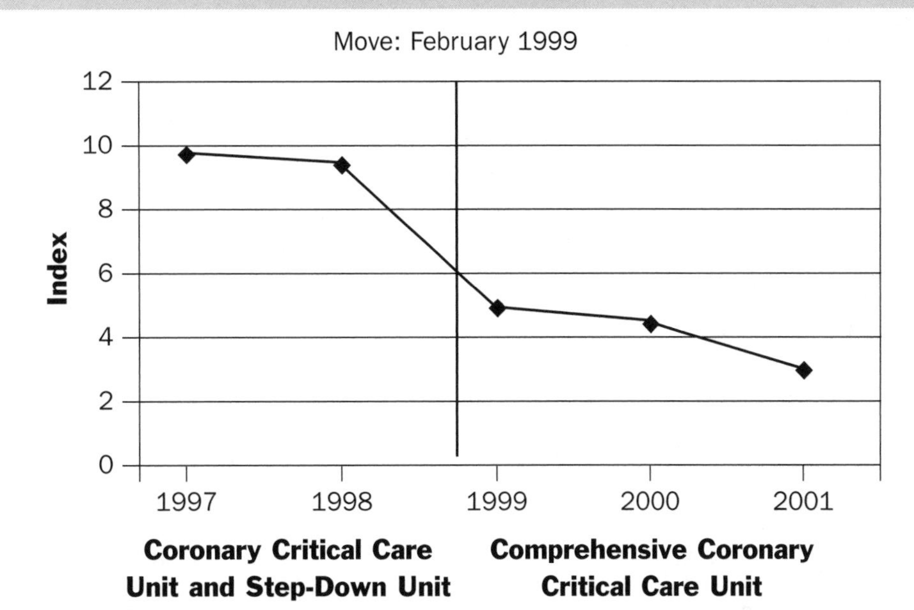

Source: Adapted from Hendrich, A., J. Fay, and A. K. Sorrells. 2004. "Effects of Acuity-Adaptable Rooms on Flow of Patients and Delivery of Care." *American Journal of Critical Care* 13 (1): 35–45.

- Medication errors reduced by 70 percent (see Figure S)
- Patient falls minimized to 2 falls per 1,000 patient days
- Patient dissatisfaction decreased by 3 percent
- Nursing efficiency improved
- Length of stay decreased

Acuity-adjustable beds represent a powerful intervention from evidence-based design. Research is ongoing to expand our knowledge of the connection between care outcomes and the physical environment. Other promising areas that are currently being explored include noise and its impact on stress (for both patients and staff) and on use of pain medication, and the effect of lighting on prescribing or dispensing medications.

WHERE TO LEARN MORE

For more information on the Transforming Care at the Bedside project and the use of acuity-adaptable beds, please see IHI's web site: http://www.ihi.org/IHI/Programs/TransformingCareAtTheBedside/.

REFERENCES

Hendrich, A., J. Fay, and A. K. Sorrells. 2004. "Effects of Acuity-Adaptable Rooms on Flow of Patients and Delivery of Care." *American Journal of Critical Care* 13 (1): 35–45.

McCarthy, M. 2004. "Healthy Design." *Lancet* 364 (9432): 405–06.

Ulrich, R., X. Quan, C. Zimring, A. Joseph, and R. Choudhary. 2004. "The Role of the Physical Environment in the Hospital of the 21st Century: A Once-in-a-Lifetime Opportunity." Report. Concord, CA: The Center for Health Design.

IDEA 10

Learn to See

The problem in life is that there is no scary music to let you know when danger is near.

Human beings, by nature, are confident in their ability to see danger coming. We put our lives in the "hands" of our eyes each time we cross a busy street or our vehicles pull out onto a busy highway. When we enter the healthcare system, we transfer this confidence from our own ability to see to others' ability to see. We trust that those charged with our care will be able to see problems developing or areas of potential danger. Because of this trust, and because of the life-or-death stakes in healthcare, it is imperative that healthcare workers really *do* see all that is to be seen.

INATTENTIONAL BLINDNESS

Healthcare, whether in hospital settings or ambulatory practices, is often a complex and risky process. To provide safe and patient-centered care, we rely on the efforts of individuals who are often rushed, under the pressure of unpredictable events, and under the stress of life-or-death situations. This pressure and stress can lead to a failure of attention often known as "inattentional blindness" (Mack and Rock 1998).

Inattentional blindness is the failure to notice unexpected events when the observer is involved in other activities, especially tasks that require attention to ▸

things that are unrelated to the unexpected event. A classic example is an exercise using a video entitled "Gorillas in Our Midst." The video shows two groups of young people passing a basketball. The "players" are divided into two teams, one wearing black shirts and the other wearing white shirts. In this exercise, observers of the video are asked to count how many players wearing white shirts successfully pass the ball to a teammate. Observers are instructed to ignore the passes made by the team wearing black. While observers generally do well at counting the number of passes made by the one team, most fail to notice a rather unusual unexpected event that occurs approximately halfway through the video: A person wearing a gorilla suit walks into the center of the frame and beats his chest, in true gorilla style, and then walks off. Astoundingly, most people who watch this video, when asked about the gorilla, respond by asking, "What gorilla?"

What is important to note about this experiment is the role the instructions play in creating inattentional blindness. Were the observers simply asked to watch the video, it is unlikely that they would fail to notice the gorilla. But by introducing a task that requires close, careful attention to another event, the observers' concentration becomes focused to a degree that hinders their observation of the unexpected event.

TASK SATURATION

Afterburner, Inc., is a leadership development and management training company that uses fighter-pilot strategies to teach top executives how to better manage their organizations. The founder of Afterburner, Jim Murphy, has identified one significant impediment to quality execution and named it "task saturation." Task saturation is just what it sounds like: It is a state of being overworked, under-resourced, and stressed. This state is familiar to just about anyone who works in a fast-paced environment, and it should be especially familiar to healthcare professionals. Murphy (2005) cites the swirl of activity in a typical hospital emergency room as an example of an environment plagued by task saturation. The danger arises when workers respond to task saturation in counterproductive ways. A common response is to shut down or to simply stop what is being done. Given the exigencies and pace of most healthcare settings, this response is probably (and hopefully) rare.

A more likely response in healthcare is the coping mechanism that Murphy calls "channelizing." Murphy defines channelizing as "focus[ing] on just one thing and ignor[ing] the others." When faced with an overwhelming number of tasks, many people decide to simply deal with just one. The choice of which one to deal with is often arbitrary, and because healthcare requires careful prioritization, this arbitrariness can be very dangerous. The problem is exacerbated when a new, unexpected task is added to an already overwhelming number of tasks. We have seen how difficult it is for overworked staff to recognize an unexpected event, but even when they do recognize such an event their response may be to ignore it and to focus instead on what they had been previously working on.

The means of combating task saturation goes right to the heart of what the idea of learning to see is about. Murphy contends that, to cope successfully with the reality of being overwhelmed by tasks, workers must learn to see how they and their colleagues usually cope. By identifying common symptoms of the dangerous coping mechanisms, workers will be able to recognize when they are failing to cope properly and to identify when others are doing the same. Equally important to combating task saturation is addressing the workload itself. Murphy argues that, in most cases, lightening the workload is not realistic; instead, he urges organizations to employ process redesign to "kill the weeds before they choke the grass."

Detecting a change in patient status or unspoken patient needs depends on the attention of overworked staff. If this change in a patient's status or needs is unrelated to what the staff is specifically paying attention to, the chances of it going unobserved increase. We need to design better processes to ensure safe and patient-centered care and to build better communication across teams.

SUGGESTIONS FOR REDESIGNING PROCESSES

An example is given after each of the following suggestions:

- Build redundant processes for observation to ensure that risks and needs are identified.

  Example: Early warning scoring systems (EWS) are a way of linking patient monitoring with visual controls to better "see" the onset of deterioration or patient distress. When routine monitors such as vital signs are charted on the EWS record, a color code alerts the staff that the patient's condition may warrant further help. Color coding and scoring of patient stability add to the information that staff can use to assess when to get input on the care. Use of the EWS has increased the number of early calls for help and decreases the number of codes on patients.

- Mid-level managers are key to creating a culture that values attention to detail and that rewards taking time for surveillance and action.

  Example: Use change-of-shift reports as an opportunity to alert the oncoming shift to potential safety hazards (e.g., "We have two patients with similar names, so we took the following steps to ensure their safety ..." or "We had a near-miss on a sleeping medication with Mrs. Smith and have changed her MAR to make the orders clearer."). Reminding the staff about safety issues at each report and at staff meetings makes visible the nurse manager's commitment to safety.

- Multidisciplinary rounds can result in a more complete assessment of patient needs, build a collaborative culture, and improve teamwork.

  Example: Multidisciplinary rounds enable all members of the care team to see the patient and to plan for next steps and changes. The unique capabilities of the various care team members yield a more complex and accurate picture of the patient's state, especially when the rounds involve the patients themselves. Teams will often add the formulation of daily goals as the team's output. Multidisciplinary rounds and daily goals have resulted in shorter lengths of stay, improvements in achieving clinical goals, and better staff and physician satisfaction.

EXAMPLE: SSM HEALTHCARE

Inattentional blindness is only one aspect of learning to see. The pace of healthcare can be so rapid that staff can run into, and be hampered by, obstacles without even noticing the obstacles themselves.

Bob Porter, executive vice president of strategy and business development at SSM Healthcare in St. Louis, Missouri, issued disposable cameras to some staff and asked them to take pictures to document barriers and frustrations in their daily work. Within 24 hours, his staff asked him for more cameras. The barriers and frustrations were everywhere, but putting the camera in front of their eyes gave them a different way to see them. As staff learned to see the barriers, they began to notice more and more. Actually asking them to take pictures, rather than just note or document the barriers and frustrations, created a different level of consciousness. In this way, the staff at SSM learned to see in new ways.

WHERE TO LEARN MORE

For information on the "Gorillas in Our Midst" video, please visit http://viscog.beckman.uiuc.edu/grafs/demos/15.html.

Learn about Failure Modes and Effects Analysis (FMEA—a systematic, proactive method for evaluating a process to identify where and how it may fail, and to assess the relative impact of different failures to identify the parts of the process that are most in need of change. Please visit http://www.ihi.org/IHI/Topics/PatientSafety/SafetyGeneral/Tools/Failure+Modes+and+Effects+Analysis+%28FMEA%29+Tool+%28IHI+Tool%29.htm.

REFERENCES

Mack, A., and I. Rock. 1998. *Inattentional Blindness*. Cambridge, MA: MIT Press.

Murphy, J. 2005. "Overcoming the Dangers of Task Saturation." *Occupational Hazards*. [Online article; retrieved 8/1/05.] http://www.occupationalhazards.com/articles/13358.

ABOUT THE AUTHORS

Maureen Bisognano is the executive vice president and chief operating officer of the Institute for Healthcare Improvement (IHI) in Cambridge, Massachusetts. She is responsible for day-to-day management of the Institute's many programs, designed to improve the delivery of healthcare. Ms. Bisognano oversees all operations, program development, and strategic planning for the Institute. In doing so, she advises healthcare leaders around the world. She is an unrelenting advocate for the needs of patients and is a passionate crusader for change.

Prior to joining IHI, Ms. Bisognano was senior vice president of the Juran Institute, where she consulted with senior management on the implementation of total quality management in healthcare settings. Before that, she served as chief executive officer of the Massachusetts Respiratory Hospital in Braintree, Massachusetts, where, as part of the National Demonstration Project, she introduced total quality management. Her accomplishments in this organization include implementation of the quality improvement program throughout all levels of the hospital, from the board of trustees to the employees. She organized and monitored quality improvement teams within the hospital to make process improvements.

Ms. Bisognano began her career in healthcare in 1973 as a staff nurse at Quincy City Hospital in Quincy, Massachusetts. She was director of nursing at Quincy City Hospital from 1981 to 1982, director of patient services from 1982 to 1986, and chief operating officer from 1986 to 1987. Ms. Bisognano holds a bachelor of science degree from the State University of New York and a master of science degree from Boston University.

Paul Plsek is an internationally recognized consultant on improvement and innovation for today's complex organizations. Before starting his own firm, he led engineering teams in Bell Labs and was director of corporate quality planning at AT&T. Mr. Plsek is the developer of the concept of DirectedCreativity™, and his work with leaders can be described as "helping organizations think better."

Mr. Plsek is the chair of innovation at the Virginia Mason Medical Center in Seattle, Washington, the codirector of the Vermont Oxford

Network's NIC/Q Neonatal Intensive Care Improvement Collaborative, and a member of several editorial boards. He is also an active investigator and contributor in research projects with the Harvard School of Public Health, the University of Vermont, AHRQ, and The Robert Wood Johnson Foundation. He is widely recognized throughout the United States and Europe for his work in quality improvement, innovation, and complexity in healthcare. His clients include The Mayo Clinic, Kaiser Permanente, and the National Health Service in Britain.

Mr. Plsek is the author of dozens of journal articles and book chapters. He has also written three books: *Quality Improvement Tools; Creativity, Innovation and Quality*; and *Edgeware: Insights from Complexity Science for Health Care Leaders*.

ACKNOWLEDGMENTS

This book is truly the result of the work of many like-minded health professionals across the United States and in Europe. You will note that few of the ideas originated with the authors and that the real helpfulness in such a compilation comes from the implementation stories, successes, and barriers described by the leaders who employ the ideas. There are thousands of healthcare leaders, many in executive offices and many on the frontlines, who deserve our thanks. We are grateful for their commitment to our mutual mission to improve the quality of healthcare.

Dan Schummers is a man of detail and eloquence. We appreciate and acknowledge that this book is his as much as ours. Dan has devoted countless hours, many phone calls, and endless edits to make this possible, all with humor and a commitment to schedule and pace. We thank you.

A special note of thanks goes to Don Berwick and every member of our amazing staff at the Institute for Healthcare Improvement. In addition, we acknowledge the vital contributions of Tom Nolan, Carol Haraden, Pat Rutherford, Andrea Kabcenell, Kevin Nolan, Roger Resar, Frank Federico, Terri Simmonds, Fran Griffin, Diane Jacobsen, Marie Schall, Allan Frankel, Kathy Duncan, Vicki Spuhler, Tom Rainey, Terry Clemmer, Peter Pronovost, Graeme Hart, Jane Justeson, Eugene Litvak, Kirk Jensen, Marilyn Rudolph, Randy Linton, Jeanne Huddleston, Lloyd Provost, John Whittington, David Calkins, Joe McCannon and the entire 100,000 Lives Campaign team, Rose Lindsay, Uma Kotagal, Jim Andersen, Tami Merryman, Jill Patak, Jim Reinertsen, Wim Schellekens, Ann Hendrich, Sarah Garrett, Jo Bibby, Lynne Maher, Helen Bevan, Lisa Godfrey-Harris, Dave Buchanan, Jennifer Phillips, Lynne Chafetz, Robert Porter, and Sister Mary Jean Ryan.

We would also like to acknowledge the essential contributions, to both the editing and writing of this book, of Jane Roessner, Frank Davidoff, and Val Weber.

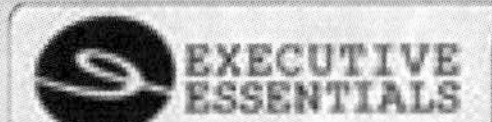

WHAT EVERY HEALTHCARE EXECUTIVE SHOULD KNOW

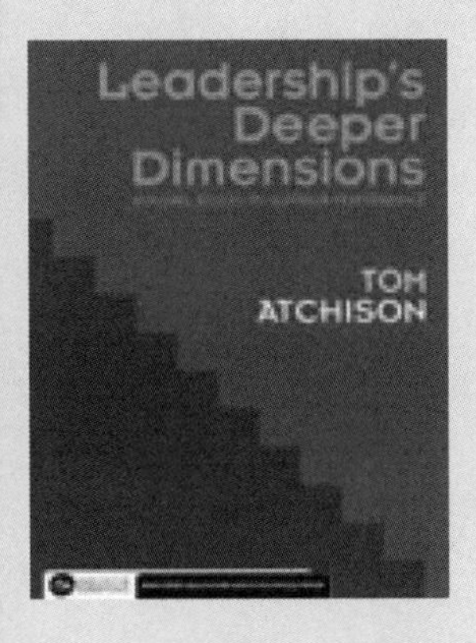

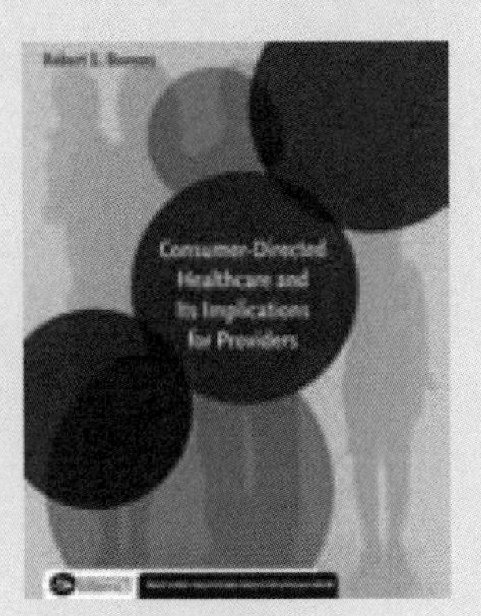

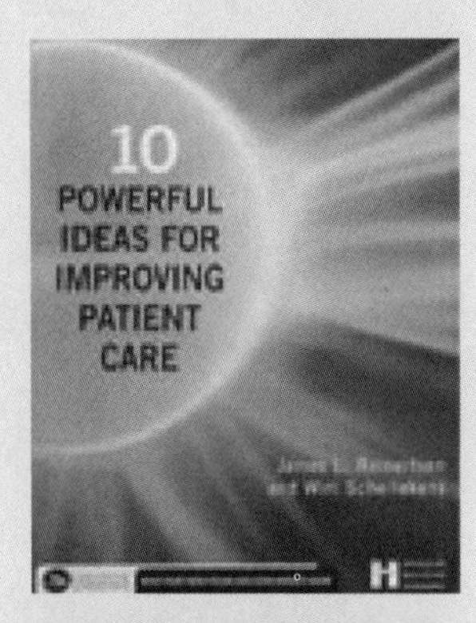

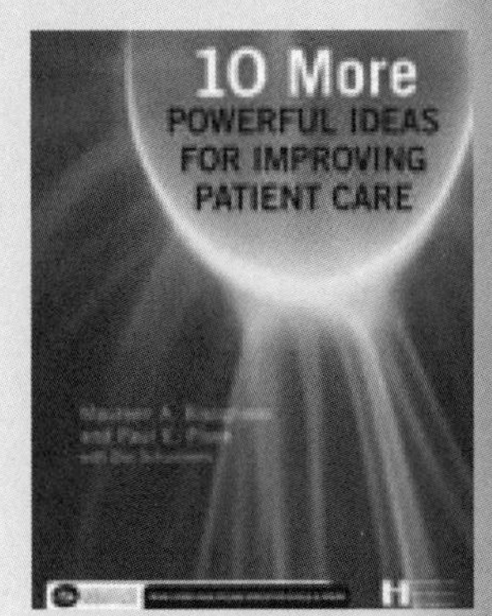

Straightforward

Executive Essentials books have a straightforward layout. Information is easy to read and find.

Focused

Executive Essentials books provide the most vital information on a topic. You won't get bogged down in superfluous details. If you do want to dig deeper into the subject, we provide a list of additional resources.

Practical

Executive Essentials books provide ready-to-use forms, charts, and checklists. Organize your work with these helpful tools.

Concise

Executive Essentials books get right to the point. Each book is 80 pages or less.

Portable

Executive Essentials books are light enough to travel with you. Learn valuable information while flying or commuting.

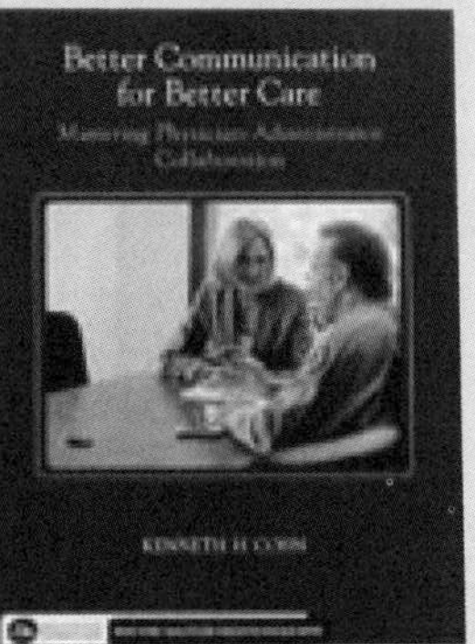

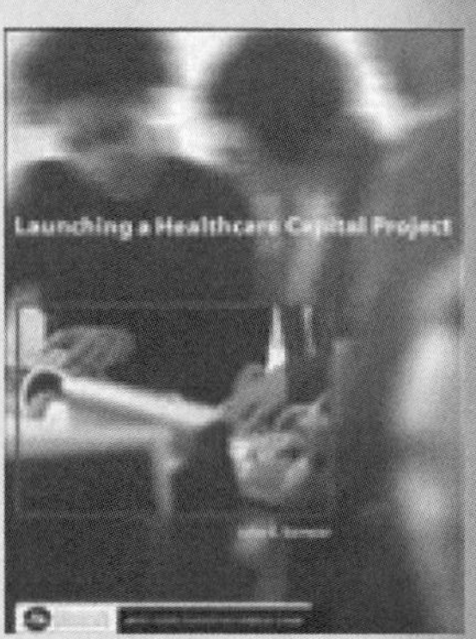

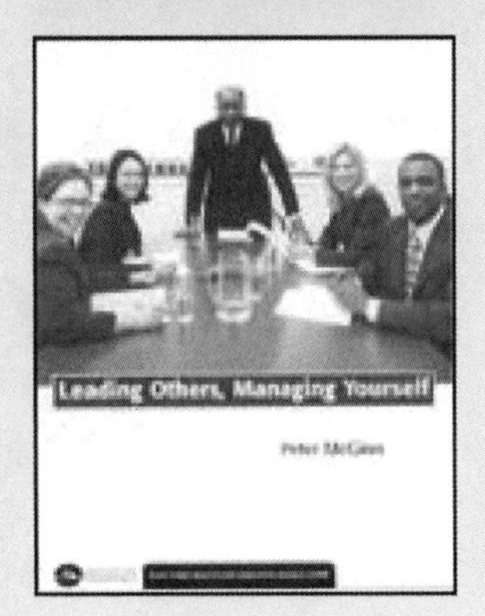

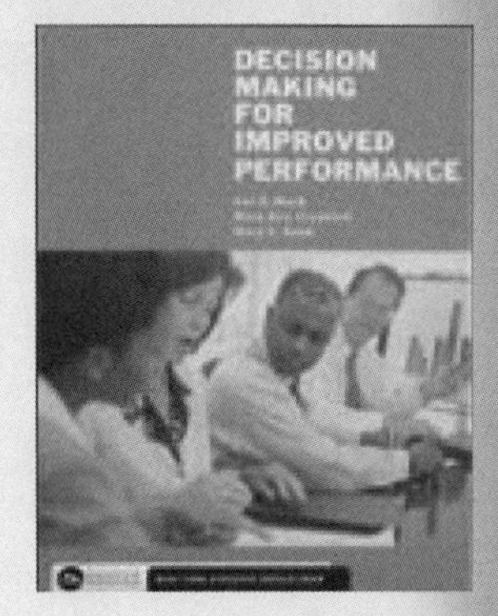

LEADING A PATIENT-SAFE ORGANIZATION

MATTHEW J. LAMBERT, III

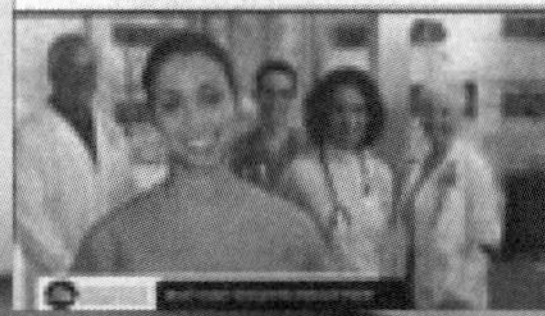

To order, call (301) 362-6905 or fax (301) 206-9789
Order online at www.ache.org/hap.cfm